THE GREAT INOCULATOR

Gavin
Weightman

THE GREAT
INOCULATOR

The Untold Story
of Daniel Sutton
and his Medical
Revolution

YALE UNIVERSITY PRESS
NEW HAVEN AND LONDON

Published with assistance from the Annie Burr Lewis Fund.

For information about this and other Yale University Press publications, please contact:
U.S. Office: sales.press@yale.edu   yalebooks.com
Europe Office: sales@yaleup.co.uk   yalebooks.co.uk

Set in Minion Pro by IDSUK (DataConnection) Ltd
Printed in Great Britain by TJ International Ltd, Padstow, Cornwall

Library of Congress Control Number: 2020938180

ISBN 978-0-300-24144-0

A catalogue record for this book is available from the British Library.

10 9 8 7 6 5 4 3 2 1

Contents

	List of Plates	vii
	Acknowledgements	ix
	Preface	xii
1	Lady Mary's Revelation	1
2	Saving the Quality	9
3	Is It Worth the Risk?	20
4	A Rural Revolution	30
5	A Most Surprising Fellow	39
6	Sutton the Parvenu	50
7	Sutton's Thunder Stolen	59
8	Sutton Misses the Boat	68
9	A Suttonian in America	79
10	An Imposter in the Family	86
11	Inoculation for the Industrious Poor	92
12	Saving the Nation	104
13	Sutton's Swan Song	112
14	Cowmania!	121
15	Jenner's Debt to Sutton	132
16	The Battle for Vaccination	145

CONTENTS

17   Sutton and Jenner: The Legacy   156

18   The Mystery of Immunity   162

Postscript: Sutton's Family   *166*

Notes   *169*

Bibliography   *176*

Index   *183*

Plates

1. Portrait of Daniel Sutton, by an unknown artist. From E.E. Wilde, *Ingatestone and the Essex Great Road with Fryerning*, Humphrey Milford, Oxford University Press, London, 1913.

2. *Lady Mary Wortley Montagu with her son, Edward Wortley Montagu, and attendants*, attributed to Jean Baptiste Vanmour, *c.* 1717. © National Portrait Gallery, London.

3. 'The Idle 'Prentice Executed at Tyburn: Industry and Idleness', by William Hogarth, 1747.

4. Portrait of Caroline Wilhelmina of Brandenburg-Ansbach when Princess of Wales, by John Smith, after Sir Godfrey Kneller, 1717. © National Portrait Gallery, London.

5. Portrait of William Wagstaffe, by an unknown artist, *c.* 1725. © National Portrait Gallery, London.

6. Portrait of James Jurin, by James Worsdale (*c.* 1692–1767). © The Royal Society.

7. Ingatestone high street, *c.* 1800. Essex Record Office.

8. Portrait of Daniel Sutton, by an unknown artist. Wellcome Collection.

9. 'Gore House, Kensington Gore', by Thomas Hosmer Shepherd, 1729–57. Royal Borough of Kensington and Chelsea.

10. Daniel Sutton's house, Maisonette. Essex Record Office.

11. Title page from a facsimile of Thomas Dimsdale's plagiaristic booklet, *The Present Method of Inoculating for the Small-pox*, Hertford, 1767.

12. Portrait of Baron Thomas Dimsdale. Essex Record Office.

13. Title page from Edward Jenner's vaccine book, *An inquiry into the causes and effects of the Variolae Vaccinae*, Sampson Low, London, 1798.

14. Statue of Edward Jenner, by William Calder Marshall, Kensington Gardens, London. Photograph from 1920–40. Wellcome Collection. Attribution 4.0 International (CC BY 4.0).

15. Engraving of Louis Pasteur in his laboratory, 1885. Wellcome Collection. Attribution 4.0 International (CC BY 4.0).

16. Title page from Daniel Sutton's book, *The Inoculator*, London, 1796.

Acknowledgements

Dr Peter Razzell first drew my attention to the remarkable success Daniel Sutton and his family of Suffolk country surgeons had as inoculators against smallpox, the deadliest of all eighteenth-century diseases. Peter was struck by the fact that this was one medical intervention that might possibly have had a measurable part to play in the rise in population in the second half of the eighteenth century. Whether it was or not, and that question is unresolved, Peter's research revealed the largely forgotten history of the origins of what later became known as vaccination. It is a subject he and I discussed many times and which, in the end, inspired this book which is dedicated to him.

I am also greatly indebted to John Smith, author of *The Speckled Monster*, a history of smallpox in England with special reference to Essex.[1] Daniel Sutton had his first practice in Ingatestone in Essex, the county in which John worked as an archivist while he was writing his book. As well as sharing his great knowledge with me, John approached Lord Rayleigh of Terling Place, Essex, for permission to quote from letters in which Bamber Gascoyne described Daniel Sutton's inoculation of his sons.[2] My thanks to Lord Rayleigh, and to John for transcribing the letters for me.

Michael Bennett, Emeritus Professor of History and Classics at the University of Tasmania, generously shared his wealth of knowledge about inoculation and vaccination with me and allowed me to read some of his recent unpublished work. Professor Bennett's account of the extraordinary career of Daniel Sutton's father-in-law Simeon Worlock opened up a chapter about which very little is known in this country. I am very grateful to him for all the help he gave me.

I discussed the life and influence of Sutton with a number of historians of medicine in the eighteenth century, notably Gareth Williams, Emeritus Professor of Medicine and Dentistry at Bristol University. Daniel Sutton's influence was discussed in Sally Irvine's 2011 East Anglia University PhD thesis on Suffolk apothecaries and surgeons and she kindly pointed me in the direction of some useful research. Rosemary Leadbetter's Oxford Brooks University thesis 'Experiencing Smallpox in Eighteenth Century England' provided valuable background information and she was kind enough to discuss her view on the Suttons.

Although eighteenth-century inoculators had no idea their success depended on stimulation of the human immune system, I thought it worth enquiring of contemporary specialists whether anything Sutton discovered might suggest he had an intuitive insight into the way in which the body fights invasive infections. I am grateful to Professor Sheena Cruickshank, Academic Lead for Public Engagement in the Lydia Becker Institute of Immunology and Inflammation at the University of Manchester for taking the time to make an assessment of Sutton's attempts at medical research as described in his book *The Inoculator*. The best that can be said is that his results were inconclusive and that he got no further than his eminent medical contemporaries in understanding the nature of smallpox. He was, simply, a brilliant empiric.

I would like to thank the staff of the London Library who were very helpful as always. So too the staff of the British Library, the Wellcome Library and the Essex Record Office for their assistance with my research. Estela Dukan in the library of the Royal College of Physicians of Edinburgh kindly sent me documents from the archive of Sir John Pringle, an admirer of Daniel Sutton.

Lastly I would like to thank Heather McCallum, who first suggested I write a book about Sutton, and Marika Lysandrou and Clarissa Sutherland at Yale University Press for seeing the book through to publication. Thanks to Sophie Richmond for her meticulous editing. Finally I would like to thank Charles Walker of United Agents for looking after my interests as always.

Preface

You will not have heard of Daniel Sutton, an eighteenth-century country surgeon, whose reputed ability to tame the most feared disease of the age won him international fame and fortune. Sutton deserves an epitaph not simply because he had undoubted success in combating illness in the heyday of medical quackery. His pioneering practice, in which he specialised in rendering patients immune to smallpox, paved the way for what later became known as *vaccination*. That innovation, introduced by Edward Jenner, was a worldwide sensation which had him later cast as the 'the father of immunology'. Jenner's fame condemned Sutton to obscurity. *The Great Inoculator* seeks to give an eighteenth-century medical revolutionary his due and to put the more famous Jenner in his place.

In Sutton's lifetime, and long after his death in 1819, medicine knew nothing of the causes of infectious diseases. Sutton himself admitted this ignorance and speculated, correctly, that until more powerful microscopes were made, which could detect minute organisms, the cause of smallpox would remain a mystery. 'Germs' were first identified as the cause of disease in the 1860s. This raises a question about the legitimacy of claiming that Daniel Sutton was a 'medical revolutionary'. We are accustomed today to believe that any 'medical breakthrough' is a result of sophisticated scientific research. Much of it is, but there has always been a place for astute observation in the advancement of medical understanding.

This is accepted in the case of Edward Jenner's discovery. He knew no more about the nature of infectious diseases than any other eighteenth-century doctor. His breakthrough came with the guess that a pox less virulent than smallpox that sometimes infected cattle could be used to protect against the human disease. Jenner invented a Latin name for cowpox which means, in effect, smallpox of the cow: *variolae vaccinae*. Very soon Jenner's inoculations became known as *vaccination* in competition with Daniel Sutton's *variolation*, in which smallpox infection itself was used for inoculation. The rivalry continued after the death of both of them until, in 1840, Suttonian inoculation was outlawed by Parliament.

It is almost impossible now to evoke for a modern readership the horrors of a smallpox epidemic. The affliction itself, in its most severe form, covered the victim from head to toe in horrid pustules which burned and then suppurated. This was what was called 'confluent' smallpox and few survived such an attack. Infants and small children were especially vulnerable, but it was thought that almost everyone in the eighteenth century was attacked by smallpox at some time in their lives. Some were lucky and got off lightly. Many others were disfigured, their faces scarred, beauty obliterated.

In his *The History of England from the Accession of James II* T.B. Macaulay wrote:

> The smallpox was always present, filling the churchyards with corpses, tormenting with constant fears all whom it had stricken, leaving on those whose lives it spared the hideous traces of its power, turning the babe into a changeling at which the mother shuddered, and making the eyes and cheeks of the bighearted maiden objects of horror to the lover.

Throughout the eighteenth century, newspapers were full of advertisements for potions which might alleviate the horrors of smallpox. There was no cure: an epidemic simply had to be endured. Each visitation of the disease in the towns and villages of Britain could spell economic disaster. Nobody wanted to come to market where smallpox was rife and the inns and shops might be deserted for weeks. When the danger had passed, the all-clear would be advertised in newspapers so that trade might resume as soon as possible.

This was the world into which Daniel Sutton was born in May 1735, in a Suffolk village, the second son of a country surgeon. He learned early in life that although there was no cure for smallpox, there was a way of getting protection from a severe attack of the disease. It was called 'engrafting' or 'inoculating', a procedure in which the surgeon with his lancet took a bit of infective matter from a smallpox pustule and rubbed it into an incision, usually made on the patient's arm or leg. The hope was that this would give rise to a mild attack of the disease which, when healed, would ensure the patient was immune for the rest of their life. It was the one redeeming feature of smallpox: observation over centuries had taught that you could not be attacked by it a second time.

The realisation that it was possible to become immune to smallpox had nothing to do with medical science. In fact, in Britain and Europe, doctors were very slow to recognise the possibility of inducing immunity by deliberate infection with the disease, the principle of all modern vaccinations. When Daniel Sutton was a young assistant surgeon, very few inoculations were performed. It was a very expensive procedure available only to the upper crust of society, which sought it chiefly to protect their children. He made it his ambition to devise a more accessible and less costly form of inoculation.

When Sutton started his own practice in 1763, there was still fierce opposition to inoculation from much of the medical profession and from the Church. Deliberately infecting a patient was anathema to most doctors, and considered sacrilegious by the clergy as it was usurping the power of God to make people ill. Shrewdly, Sutton advertised for a clergyman to see to the spiritual needs of his patients and to give a blessing to his practice. The Revd Robert Houlton, one of the chaplains to the Earl of Ilchester, took the job, in Ingatestone in Essex, where Sutton had his pioneer practice, and became, in effect, Sutton's public relations officer.

Houlton preached a sermon in favour of inoculation and, in 1766, had it published with this dedication:

> Ever indebted will these kingdoms be to the late honourable Lady Mary Wortley Montague [sic] ... for the great and noble blessing, Inoculation. Thousands of subjects, the tender husband, the affectionate wife, fond parents and pious children engrave her name in deep characters on their hearts and will record it forever with gratitude and praise.[1]

Likewise, Daniel Sutton recognised that the foundations of his fortune were laid by this courageous and enterprising aristocratic lady a quarter of a century before he was born. Who was she and why was she worthy of such adulation?

1

Lady Mary's Revelation

Lady Mary Wortley Montagu was born into an aristocratic family in 1689, a daughter of Evelyn Pierrepont who was created Marquess of Dorchester in 1706 and later, Duke of Kingston upon Hull. From an early age Lady Mary was determined to educate herself, which she did secretly, as her father did not think it proper for a lady to trouble herself with serious topics. After her mother died when Mary was just 3 years old, a grandmother cared for her until she died, after which she was cared for by her father. The family home was Thorsby Hall in Nottinghamshire, with a well-stocked library where, as Lady Mary put it, she 'stole' her education. While it was assumed she was reading romantic novels, she taught herself Latin and began to write poetry.

She was single-minded and wilful, refusing to marry the man her father thought suitable and thereby losing her dowry. Instead she eloped with Edward Wortley Montagu, whom she married in Salisbury in August 1712. She lived in the countryside for three years during which time her son Edward was born. After George I came to the throne in 1714, the Wortley Montagus moved to London, where Lady Mary became a glittering society figure, hobnobbing with the royal family. She also became friends with a number of writers, including Alexander Pope.

In 1715, at the height of her notoriety in London society, she was struck down by an attack of malignant smallpox. It was assumed for a while she would not survive, but she pulled through, although scarred by the loss of her much admired eyebrows. A brother who also suffered an attack, died of the disease when doctors had assured Lady Mary that he had a good chance of survival. From that time onwards she had a very low opinion of the higher echelons of the medical profession.

When her husband, Wortley Montagu, was appointed ambassador to Turkey, Lady Mary joined him, enduring a long, but fascinating, journey overland, taking her 3-year-old son Edward with her. A Scottish surgeon, Charles Maitland, accompanied them as the embassy doctor. They stayed first in Adrianople, where, for the first time, Lady Mary became aware of the practice of 'transplanting' the smallpox. The simplicity and effectiveness of it seemed miraculous. Elderly women made punctures in the arms of children and rubbed in infectious smallpox matter. The symptoms of the disease as it developed were light, and when the few pustules died away there were no pock marks. She wrote to her friend Sarah Chiswell 'A propos of distempers, I am going to tell you a thing that I am sure will make you wish yourself here. The small-pox, so fatal, and so general amongst us, is here entirely harmless by the invention of *ingrafting*, which is the term they give it.'

After describing how the operation was performed she continued: 'I am patriot enough to take pains to bring this useful invention into fashion in England; and I should not fail to write to some of our doctors very particularly about it, if I knew any one of them that I thought had virtue enough to destroy such a considerable branch of their revenue for the good of mankind.'[1]

Constantinople was exciting and inspiring. The ambassador's residence was a rented palace in Pera, a district high above the Golden Horn with a view over it. It teemed with officials and staff, and from her window Lady Mary could see 'the port, the city, the seraglio [harem] and the distant hills of Asia; perhaps all together [*sic*] the most beautiful prospect in the world'.[2]

She was pregnant and gave birth in Constantinople to a girl, Mary. Dr Maitland was in attendance and so too, though not necessarily to see her through her pregnancy, was Emanuel Timoni, a doctor who had trained in Italy and England but who was resident in Turkey. The ambassador had engaged Timoni, the son of a dragoman, a translator and mediator between the West and the Ottoman rulers. He had written (in Latin originally) a favourable account of the practice of 'transplanting', which had been published in 1716 in the *Transactions of the Royal Society*, a year before Lady Mary arrived in Constantinople.

Though Maitland does not mention Timoni, it seems likely that it was he who influenced Lady Mary when she decided to get her son Edward inoculated. Certainly Timoni's view on the safety and success of inoculation in Turkey must have been reassuring for Dr Maitland when Lady Mary put him on the spot by asking him to find one of the elderly Greek ladies who performed the operation so that her son Edward could be engrafted in the same way as Turkish children.

Maitland recalled:

the Ambassador's ingenious Lady, who had been at some Pains to satisfie her Curiosity in this Matter, and had made some useful Observations on the Practice, was so thoroughly convinced of the Safety of it, that She resolv'd to submit her only Son to it, a very hopeful Boy of about Six Years of Age: She first of all order'd me to find out a fit Subject to take the Matter from; and then sent for an old Greek Woman, who had practis'd this Way a great many years.[3]

Before he was prepared to carry out Lady Mary's wishes, Maitland wrote that he first wanted to satisfy himself that 'engrafting was safe'.

He concluded that it was not only safe but an ingenious means of protecting against smallpox: 'My Enquiry chiefly turn'd upon two or three Particulars, which, I thought, could I be well satisfied in, would go a great way towards convincing me of the mighty Advantages and Safety of the Method, and resolving my greatest Scruples and Difficulties against it.'

Maitland wanted to feel sure that Turkish smallpox was much the same as that back home, and that engrafting would not be damaging or dangerous to the young boy. In fact, he concluded: 'I could not forbear admiring the very great Sagacity of the Men who first invented this Method; and the laudable and diligent Observation of them too, who so carefully practis'd it themselves, and so faithfully convey'd it to their Neighbours.'[4]

Nevertheless, it was with some trepidation that he went about carrying out Lady Mary's wishes. 'After a good deal of Trouble and Pains,' he recalled:

I found a proper Subject, and then the good Woman went to work; but so awkwardly by the shaking of her Hand, and put the Child to so much Torture with her blunt and rusty Needle, that I pitied his Cries . . . and therefore Inoculated the other Arm with my own Instrument, and with so little Pain to him, that he did not in the least complain of it. The Operation took in both Arms, and succeeded perfectly well.[5]

Three days after the inoculation bright spots appeared on Edward's face and then disappeared. After a week he was thirsty and hot, after which, as Maitland recalled, the 'smallpox came out fair'. He had more than 100 pustules which fell off after a while leaving no scars. The boy did not suffer any other illness. His mother was overjoyed and decided to have her infant daughter inoculated. Lady Mary would have had this second inoculation carried out in Constantinople but was concerned for the girl's nurse, who had not had smallpox. As it happened, her husband was recalled to London sooner than anticipated and the family and Dr Maitland followed.

It was one thing to have her son inoculated in the exotic world of Constantinople where the procedure was commonplace: it was quite another to risk it in London. Lady Mary was well aware of this and planned to have her daughter inoculated secretly. But Charles Maitland pleaded to have witnesses for fear of damaging his professional reputation. This was the first ever inoculation carried out in Britain, or anywhere in Europe, by a professional, and Lady Mary and Maitland knew very well that they were laying themselves open to fierce criticism.

In spring 1721, Maitland recorded his anxiety in an account he wrote of this momentous event in medical history:

> This Noble Lady sent for me last April, and when I came, she told me, she was now resolved to have her Daughter Inoculated, and desir'd me forthwith to find out Matter for the Purpose. I . . . pray'd, that any two Physicians, whom they thought fit, might be call'd, not only to consult the Health and Safety of the Child, but likewise to be Eyewitnesses of the Practice, and contribute to the Credit and Reputation of it. This indeed was at first deny'd me, it may be, out of a Design to keep it secret, or lest it should come to nothing.[6]

It was customary to prepare a patient for medical treatment with blood letting and laxatives, in the belief that somehow there would be a 'cleansing of the blood'. Maitland wrote that he decided to do without this elaborate preliminary and to go ahead once he had found what he called 'proper matter', by which he meant live infection from the pustule of a smallpox sufferer. It was ten days after the incision that the smallpox appeared and there was a period of anxiety as feverishness was accompanied by the appearance of the pocks or pustules.

I ingrafted it in both Arms, after the usual Manner; the Child was neither blooded nor purg'd before, nor indeed was it necessary, considering the clean Habit of Body, and the very cool, regular Diet she had ever been kept to from her Infancy. She continued easie and well, without any sensible Alteration . . . till the tenth Night, when she was observ'd to be a little hot and Feverish . . . and the Small Pox began next Morning to appear, which was indeed some two Days later than usual, by reason of the uncommon Discharge of Matter at the Incisions from the Beginning.[7]

The fewer pocks the less virulent the attack. Lady Mary's daughter was barely troubled, as Maitland recorded:

Three learned Physicians of the College were admitted, one after another, to visit the young Lady; they are all Gentlemen of Honour, and will on all Occasions declare, as they have hitherto done, that they saw Miss Wortley playing about the Room, cheerful and well, with the Small Pox rais'd upon her; and that in a few Days after she perfectly recover'd of them. Several Ladies, and other Persons of Distinction, visited also this young Patient, and can attest the Truth of this Fact.[8]

A Dr Keith, who was a witness to young Mary's recovery, was impressed enough to ask Maitland to inoculate his 6-year-old son. However, Lady Mary's recollection of this momentous occasion was rather different as she made clear in her private correspondence.

Lord Wharncliffe, editor of Lady Mary's letters wrote:

But what said Lady Mary of the actual fact and the actual time? Why, that the four great physicians deputed by government to watch the progress of her daughter's inoculation, betrayed not only such incredulity as to its success, but such an unwillingness to have it succeed, such an evident spirit of rancour and malignity, that she never cared to leave the child alone with them one second lest it should in some secret way suffer from their interference.

The recollections of her daughter, who later became Lady Bute, are of the keenness of those families risking the inoculation of their children to ask for her advice, but more generally a suspicion of her and her mother. According to Wharncliffe: 'From six years old upwards, Lady Bute could see the significant shrugs of the nurses and servants, and observe the looks of dislike they cast at her mother.'

Lady Mary's attempt to introduce to Britain what she believed was a miraculous preventive of the ravages of smallpox looked at first as if it might have failed. In fact it has been argued by one distinguished academic that her historical importance in introducing this medical innovation has been exaggerated, and she should be 'taken down a peg'.[9] The innovation would have happened sooner or later, it is argued, because the time was ripe and inoculation was introduced to Boston in New England at more or less the same time without any influence from Lady Mary. There were accounts from two distinguished doctors of the success of inoculation in Turkey before Lady Mary first encountered it. Many merchants and travellers had noted the practice.

Perhaps Lady Mary's importance has been exaggerated. However, her experience was not lost on Daniel Sutton, who, it will be seen was very much influenced by Lady Mary's account of the primitive 'folk' practice of inoculation when he came to devise his own 'Suttonian' method. And it was surely Lady Mary's brave example in having her daughter inoculated which caught the attention of Princess Caroline, daughter-in-law of George I.

Caroline had three young daughters. Fearing for their safety, she considered following Lady Mary's example, but she was not so bold as to risk this untried and potentially dangerous procedure. In consultation with doctors appointed to the Royal Court, she sponsored an extraordinary medical experiment to take place in London's notorious Newgate Gaol. It was this bold – and by today's standards quite unethical – trial of the safety of inoculation that first introduced the novel procedure to the public. The fierce disagreements it gave rise to in the eighteenth century are still with us today.

2

Saving the Quality

Some newspapers got hold of the proposed Newgate experiment but did not know quite what to make of it. The *Daily Journal* of 17 June 1721 attempted to explain why the upper crust might be prepared to deliberately infect themselves with 'the distemper'. What the readers would have made of it is impossible to say:

> A project is on foot for inoculating the smallpox by incision from one person to another in order to save the Lives of the Quality, who are willing, it seems, to compound with the Distemper, by taking the best sort of these Pox gratis, and thereby prevent their having the worst kind, which are called the Confluent or Mortal pox; the Experiment is to be tried upon two of the condemned malefactors in Newgate who for undergoing the Operation are to have their pardons.[1]

The experiment Princess Caroline sponsored, and which was overseen by Sir Hans Sloane and other royal medics, required condemned prisoners in Newgate to agree to be inoculated in return for a pardon granted by King George I. As one newspaper put it, if you were going to be hanged anyway, risking inoculation was not a bad bargain, implying that anyone who was *not* destined for the gallows might do well not to risk it.

Six volunteers were found, apparently without difficulty: three women and three men, of whom five were sentenced to death and a sixth to transportation. Their names and histories and the reasons they were to be sent to the gallows were apparently of no great interest to the newspapers. What little we know of them can only be gleaned from the trial records of the Old Bailey, London's Central Criminal Court. Surprisingly perhaps, none of those seeking a pardon were murderers or guilty of manslaughter.

Manacled in her cell in Newgate Prison awaiting execution on the gallows at Tyburn was Elizabeth Harrison, just 19 years old who had been working as a servant in the home of a wealthy family. She was caught embezzling 62 guineas from her employer. Any theft valued at over £5 carried the death penalty and she had no defence. She pleaded guilty at the Old Bailey on 19 April 1721. Once she volunteered to be a Newgate guinea pig, she knew she had escaped a grim ritual which was familiar to all Londoners in the eighteenth century.

A tumbril, the execution wagon, would take her with fellow condemned convicts through excited and often unruly crowds along a fixed route of more than 2 miles from Newgate to the three-cornered gallows at Tyburn, on the outskirts of London, roughly where Marble Arch is today. Along the way the condemned were allowed their last drinks of gin or beer. Once she reached Tyburn, Elizabeth would be given a moment to confess her sins to the crowd, who might pelt her with mud and rubbish. She would be blindfolded, and perhaps hooded, her hands tied behind her back and a noose put around her neck.

Thieves and highwaymen often showed bravado on their way to the gallows, as the tumbril moved through the crowds along what would later be Oxford Street. But when they were close to the hangman's noose they nearly all collapsed with fear and had to be supported in the tumbril before the horses were whipped into action. The condemned were left dangling, still alive, dying slowly from strangulation. Family and friends, if she had any there, might grab Elizabeth's legs and pull down to break her neck and hasten the end of her misery.

Once she agreed to take part in the inoculation trial, Elizabeth not only escaped this horrible death, she was afforded privileged treatment in Newgate. It was reasoned that an unhealthy guinea pig might give inoculation a bad name. So Elizabeth was moved to an 'airy' part of the prison, where she was prescribed a special diet ordered by the doctors. In the summer of 1721, five other prisoner-volunteers joined her in the 'airy cells' at Newgate.

Ann Tompion, aged twenty-five, had robbed a woman of her silk purse. Tompion and her husband were in a boat on the Thames at Temple Stairs when they came across a woman calling out 'Two Pence to Pepper Alley' and offered to take her. It was in the boat that Ann lifted the woman's purse, and her husband rowed away, leaving their passenger penniless. They were tracked down by their victim who wore a 'Red Riding Hood' cloak as a disguise to identify them. Unaccountably, Mr Tompion was acquitted. Ann's death sentence was 'respited' when she 'pleaded her belly' and was found to be 'quick with child' by a jury of matrons. That was in October 1720, so her child would have been born before the Newgate experiment began and her death sentence could no longer be postponed.

John Alcock, 20 years old, a Londoner from St Martin-in-the-Fields, had been working for a family in Berkshire when he took the wife's horse at night, along with a set of silver spurs, and made off with his employer's silk handkerchief, muslin cravat and Holland shirt. It was not long before he was tracked down and the horse retrieved: but not the silver spurs, which he said he had sold. He and Richard Evans, aged nineteen, who confessed to stealing a riding hood and fourteen yards of Persian silk from a shop-keeper and giving them to an accomplice to take to a pawn-broker, were also facing the gallows.

Poor Mary North, who was the oldest of the condemned at thirty-six, claimed that she suffered from mental illness and, according to accounts of her behaviour at the Old Bailey, and later in the condemned cell, she had 'lunatic' episodes, where she ranted and raved. She had been convicted of stealing in March 1720 and transported to the West Indies. The following year she was back in London having returned illegally, an offence which carried the death penalty. This harsh law had been in place only a year in 1721 and, according to Newgate records, those caught by it could not believe they would be hung for breaking it.

One other prisoner who volunteered was John Cauthrey, aged twenty-five, who had stolen wigs and other goods from his employer and attempted to sell them. His sentence had been transportation, which at that time meant seven years exile in the colonies, often Jamaica or the small island of Nevis.

The experiment had been proposed to the king by Sir Hans Sloane, one of the royal doctors (he attended Queen Anne in 1712 and later George II) and approval was given on the understanding that it might benefit mankind. It was of intense interest to all the senior medical men in London, though there were some who disapproved. There was one practical problem: none of them was familiar with the 'engrafting' procedure. The only surgeon who had any experience at all was Charles Maitland. He was reluctant to get involved, but in the end agreed to be the inoculator at a time when he was looking forward to a quiet retirement. Mr Maitland's *Newgate Journal*, included in his *Account of Inoculating the Smallpox*, published in 1722, gives a day-by-day account of the reactions of each of the prisoners to inoculation of the smallpox:

August 1721. In Obedience to their Royal Highnesses Commands, I performed the Operation of Inoculating the Small Pox, on Six condemned Criminals at Newgate . . . betwixt the Hours of 9 and 10 in the Morning, I made Incisions in both Arms and the right Leg of all the Six.

10th and 11th. *Thursday* and *Friday*, They all sleep well, dress, and walk about all day, and are hungry for their Food . . .

12th *Saturday* . . . suspecting the Matter ingrafted to have been defective and languid . . . I search'd for fresh Matter, and having found it in Christ's Hospital, about 6 a Clock at Night I made new Incisions in each Arm of five of them, and ingrafted it as before. I had no Matter left for the sixth, Evans.

13th *Sunday*. Morning, these five complain all of Pain in both Arms: Having taken off the Dressings, I find all the first Incisions inflamed and fester'd, but without any Sickness in the Patients . . .

14th *Monday*. Morning, red Spots and Flushings appear on all the five; but most of all on Mary North, especially about her Face, Neck, and Breast: And so likewise on Ann Tompion: But without any Sickness, Head-ach, or Thirst . . .

15th *Tuesday*. The same Spots and Flushings appear fresh in the Morning; but turn paler and darker towards Night . . . It is here to be observed, That the sixth, viz. Richard Evans . . . has had no manner of Pain, Heat, or Inflammation [he did not tell the doctors he had had smallpox and was therefore already immune].

16th *Wednesday*. They all continue much as before, only their Incisions begin to discharge a thick, purulent Matter. Anne Tompion has a large yellow Pustule on the bending of her Thigh, and another on the outside of her right, Arm, like Small Pox: And John Alcock has more fresh Pustules appearing on his Face and Arms; having had a slight Febricula (fever) in the Night, with disturb'd Water. And John Cawthery has a large yellow Pustule on his left Cheek, and several small ones on his Face.

17th *Thursday*. The said Alcock has these Pustules appearing now fairly, with a yellow digested Matter, and red Bottoms, and a great many of them, but without Sickness. Ann Tompion has the same yellow Pustules on her right Arm and Thigh, with other fresh ones struck out about her Chin and Mouth.

18th *Friday*. Alcock's Small Pox appear still fair and yellow, but fuller and larger, with a bright red round them. All the others much the same, with their Incisions running.

19th *Saturday*. Last Night, this Alcock unaccountably pricks and opens all the Pustules he could come at with a Pin; which occasions them to fall and crust sooner . . . It is here to be noted, that tho' he has had by much the greatest Number of Pustules or Small Pox upon him, yet the second Time he was touch'd in one Arm only . . .

20th and 21st. *Sunday* and *Monday*, All of them continue as before . . . I believe them to be, in all respects, as safe from any future Infection as Alcock,

22nd and 23rd. *Tuesday* and *Wednesday*, All of them continue well; and their Incisions cease running, and dry up apace.[2]

Finally the male prisoners were 'purged', that is given an emetic, and watched over until all the symptoms of smallpox had gone. The three women, it was discovered, had their periods simultaneously and could not be purged. However, it was not until 6 September, nearly a month after they were inoculated that 'they were all dismiss'd to their several Counties and Habitations'.

Dr Maitland was greatly relieved and expressed his surprise and happiness at the success of the experiment:

it is particularly remarkable in this whole Affair that tho' there was not the least encouraging or favourable Circumstance attending it before the Operation; yet after it, nothing in any sort dangerous or unsuccessful did happen: Although no Art, nor stimulating Medicine, was made Use of to promote the Eruptions; not so much as to oblige the Patients to keep their Bed; the whole having been left to Nature, assisted by a strict and regular Diet.[3]

The Newgate trial was a success, as far as Maitland was concerned, and he was asked to inoculate the children of some aristocratic families. Yet, most of the medical profession disapproved. In 1722, the apothecary at Christ's Hospital in London, Isaac Massey, published a pamphlet entitled *A short and plain account of inoculation – with some remarks on the main arguments made use of to recommend the practice, by Mr Maitland and others*. He took a dig at Maitland:

I remember Mr Maitland at *Child's Coffee-House*, when this practice was just begun at Newgate, was as confident and positive of the success and security proposed by it, as if he had had Twenty Years Experience without any miscarriage, which made those who heard him justly suspect, he was more concerned for the *employ* than the *success* of it, and I could not but take Notice afterwards with what united Force and Zeal the practice was pushed on from its admission into the Royal Palace.

William Wagstaffe, a physician at Barts in London and a Fellow of the Royal College of Physicians, had been one of the eminent doctors who witnessed the inoculation of the Newgate Prisoners. He was not impressed unconvinced of the efficacy or value of an experiment he regarded as lacking any scientific or rational justification. In a letter to a fellow doctor published in 1722, Wagstaffe wrote:

Tho' the *Fashion* of Inoculating the Small Pox has so far prevailed, as to be admitted into the greatest Families, yet I entirely concur with You in Opinion, that, till we have fuller Evidence of the Success of it, both with regard to the security of the operation, and the certainty of preventing the like Distemper from any other cause, Physicians at least, who of all Men ought to be guided in their judgements chiefly by experience, should not be over hasty in encouraging the practice, which does not seem as yet sufficiently supported either by Reason, or by Fact.[4]

What Wagstaffe found especially galling was the fact that inoculation had been imported to England from an uncivilised country where it was practised by people with no medical knowledge.

The Country from whence we derived this Experiment, will have but very little influence on our Faith, if we consider either the Nature of the Climate, or the Capacity of the Inhabitants; and Posterity perhaps will scarcely be brought to believe that an experiment practiced [*sic*] only by a few *Ignorant Women* [his italics] amongst an illiterate and unthinking People, should of a sudden, and upon slender experience, so far obtain in one of the Politest Nations in the World, as to be received into the *Royal Palace.*

Privately, Lady Mary was furious with the medical profession for what she regarded as their blind prejudice against inoculation but, by convention at the time, she could only express her exasperation anonymously. In September 1722 the *Flying Post* newspaper published an article with the title 'A plain account of the inoculating of the Small Pox at Constantinople' and attributed to 'A Turky-Merchant [*sic*]'. It began:

16

> Out of compassion to the numbers abused and deluded by the knavery and ignorance of physicians I am determined to give a true account of the manner of inoculating the small pox as practised at Constantinople with constant success and without any ill consequences whatever. I shall sell no drugs and take no fees could I persuade people of the safety and reasonableness of this easy operation.[5]

This is the version she sent to the newspaper: it was altered for publication where 'knavery and ignorance' was of 'some persons' not physicians.

Lady Mary gave a graphic description of the way she had seen engrafting practised in Turkey. The smallpox matter was ideally taken from a fit young person who had the best sort of smallpox:

> The old nurse, who is the general surgeon upon this occasion at Constantinople, takes it in a nutshell, which holds enough to infect fifty people, contrary to the infamous practice in some places [she had written 'here'] which is to fill the blood with such a quantity of matter, as often endangers the life and never fails to make the distemper more violent than it need be.

The Newgate experiment for 'saving the lives of the Quality' only served to stir controversy over the value of inoculation and it did not persuade Princess Caroline or her medical advisers that she should follow Lady Mary's example. A question raised by Wagstaffe, the Barts physician fiercely opposed to inoculation, was whether or not the Newgate prisoners had suffered from 'genuine' smallpox. If they had not, they would still not be immune to the true disease. This was a worrying question for Princess Caroline and her royal doctors. A further experiment was needed. Together, Sir Hans Sloane and Dr Steigerthal, Physician to the King, contrived another role for the hapless Elizabeth Harrison before she could enjoy her freedom. They asked Charles Maitland to arrange for her to be exposed to a smallpox sufferer in such a way that she would not escape infection if she were not genuinely immune. He reported:

> I first employ'd her [Harrison] as Nurse to a Servant Maid, very ill and full of the continued-distinct Kind of the Small Pox, in the House of Mrs. Moss, in Christ's Hospital Buildings at Hertford, whom she attended during the whole Course of the Disease. This Maid had hardly recover'd, when one of the Boys, about ten Years Old, of the said Hospital, was also seiz'd with the very same Sort; I oblig'd her to lie every Night in the same Bed with this Boy, and to attend him constantly from the first Beginning of the Distemper to the very End: And thus she continued for Six Weeks together, without Intermission, or feeling any the least Head-Ach or other Disorder; tho', indeed, I once saw some Heats and little Pimples upon her, as Nurses commonly have under such Confinements. There's no Ground to question this Fact, being attested by a Cloud of Witnesses.[6]

Whether or not it was this ordeal that drove Harrison back to her old life, inoculation against smallpox proved to provide no protection against the criminal impulse. The Old Bailey archives record that in February 1722, Harrison and a friend went drinking in London with an eye to relieving a man of his money. Their intended victim, a John Barter, told the court that between ten and eleven at night he met the prisoners, who persuaded him to go to a brandy shop. Harrison called for Geneva (gin) and 'grew very familiar with his breeches', as he put it. When he felt her hand in his pocket he imagined he was being invited 'upstairs'. After she had spurned his advances he realised she had stolen most of his money. By that summer of 1722, Harrison was at sea, en route to the West Indies where she would at least be immune from frequent smallpox epidemics which ravaged the islands. Two other Newgate volunteers, Alcock and Evans, soon followed after being convicted at the Old Bailey of further offences.

As far as Princess Caroline was concerned, the Newgate experiment, whatever the consequences for Elizabeth and the other volunteers, was not conclusive. Though none of the five who had not previously had smallpox died or were seriously disfigured, that was a small sample on which to judge the risk of inoculation. She wanted more evidence before she dared to risk the lives of her daughters.

3

Is It Worth the Risk?

The *London Gazette* of 6–10 March 1722 reported:

> Since the Experiment made some time ago upon several criminals in Newgate, their Royal Highnesses the Prince and Princess of Wales, being desirous for a Confirmation of the Safety and Ease of this Practice, that a further Experiment should be made, six persons more had the small-pox inoculated on them . . . which has succeeded very well, the small pox being broke out in most of them.[1]

The newspaper added that these guinea pigs had been put on public display: 'the Curious may be further satisfied by a Sight of those persons at Mr Forster's House in Marlborough Court at the upper end of Poland Street and Berwick Street in Soho where Attendance is given every Day from Ten till Twelve before Noon, and from Two till Four in the Afternoon'. These 'persons' were orphans in the care of Westminster. We do not know their names nor whether they were offered any kind of inducement. In fact they may not have known what was happening to them because inoculation was something quite unknown among the poor in London and all other towns and villages in the 1720s.

Though the orphans enjoyed a complete recovery, Princess Caroline still hesitated to subject her daughters to the same novel procedure. For further assurance she asked Sir Hans Sloane for advice. He was cautious, telling the princess, as he recalled later, that inoculation seemed to 'secure people from the great dangers attending the distemper in the natural way'. Princess Caroline was not happy with such a vague and non-committal recommendation. Sloane recalled: 'The princess then asked me if I would dissuade her from it: to which I made the answer, that I would not, in a matter so likely to be such an advantage.'

At this, Princess Caroline decided that she would go ahead with it and ordered Sloane to speak to the king. Sloane wrote: 'I told his majesty my opinion that it was impossible to be certain but that raising such a commotion in the blood, there might happen dangerous accidents not foreseen.'[2] He said that King George told him boldly that the same risk was taken with any medical procedure. Bowing to his majesty's common sense, Sir Hans agreed and the inoculation of two of the princesses, Amelia and Carolina, went ahead without any misfortune. Dr Maitland supervised the operation which was performed by the King's surgeon, Claude Amyand.

Thereafter, the inoculation of royal and aristocratic children was covered in daily bulletins by newspapers. When Princess Caroline chose to have her youngest son Prince William Augustus inoculated, the *Daily Post* reported on 13 May 1723: 'On Saturday last Mr Amyand, a noted surgeon, inoculated the smallpox at Leicester House, upon the young Prince William Augustus, aged 13 months. Sir Hans Sloane and other eminent physicians being present.' Three days later he was reported well with no symptoms and looked after by four servants who ensured that the infant did not have any contact with the youngest princess. On 17 May the smallpox pustules appeared.

News that Prince William had recovered and was out of danger came on 1 June. He 'took the air' on 10 June 1723 and the *London Journal* commented: 'The Royal Family's approval of this Method is what induced several of the Nobility to give into it; for since the operation hath been performed on the young Prince, the Lord Darnley hath had three of his children inoculated for the same distemper.'

William survived to take the title Duke of Cumberland and earn the nickname 'Butcher Cumberland' for the part he played in the brutal suppression of rebel Scottish highlanders in 1745–6. However, there were other privileged infants who developed full-blown smallpox from their inoculation and did not survive. These cases were also reported in the newspapers:

Wednesday morning dy'd Miss Rolt between nine and ten years of age, daughter of the late Edward Rolt of Sacomb in the County of Hertford Esq; Member of Parliament for Chippenham in the county of Wilts; she was inoculated for the small pox nine weeks before but had been in great misery and torture almost ever since to the day of her death by a humour that broke out in several parts of her body and caused between 20 and 30 sores that could not be healed; so that this once, pretty creature and a fondling of the family, as we are informed, became a most melancholy object, which may justly cause matter of sad reflection to her relatives and (as one would think) to the operators in this new practice introduced among us.[3]

In this case, and a number of other tragedies which were reported in the newspapers, the name of the surgeon who carried out the inoculation was not mentioned. It was impossible to judge the dangers of 'this new practice' because the technique of inoculation was not described or disclosed. Lady Mary, in her diatribe in the *Flying Post*, believed doctors were 'murdering' their patients (her term was censored by the editor) because the potions and purges they used only served to weaken the latter. She went as far to suggest that the medical profession was deliberately making inoculation dangerous to protect their incomes, which came from treating the disease:

> The miserable gashes that they give people in the arms may endanger the loss of them, and the vast quantity they throw in of that infectious matter may possibly give them the worst kind of small pox, and the cordials that they pour down their throats may increase the fever to such a degree as may put an end to their lives. After some few more sacrifices of this kind it may be hoped this terrible design against the revenue of the College may be entirely defeated, and those worthy members receive two guineas a day as before, of the wretches that send for them in that distemper.[4]

For those families contemplating inoculation for their children or themselves, there was precious little evidence on which to make an informed decision. Half a dozen convicts and a few orphans had clearly survived unharmed. But there had been deaths. The big question for patients and doctors was: 'Is it worth the risk?'

It is a question still asked today by those sceptical of the safety of vaccination when the risks are demonstrably minimal. In the 1720s, when the value of inoculation was fiercely disputed nobody could say what the risks were. Charles Maitland, the pioneer inoculator of Lady Mary's children, wrote a strongly worded refutation of the argument by eminent doctors, such as William Wagstaffe, that inoculation was no safer than catching smallpox in the natural way. Wagstaffe had argued that because the Newgate prisoners had had relatively mild attacks it was 'not true smallpox' but some other disease. Maitland's rejoinder was that inoculated smallpox *was* usually milder than the infection caught naturally. The choice was stark: go for inoculation and hope to gain immunity, or risk catching the disease 'naturally' and risk death.

However, there was precious little evidence to go on as there had been so few inoculations after the Newgate experiment. Few doctors would risk their reputation and livelihood by attempting it. An exception was Thomas Nettleton, a physician whose practice was in Halifax in Yorkshire, in the north of England. Just before the princesses were inoculated he had been so horrified by the ravages of an outbreak of smallpox in Halifax that he felt compelled to give inoculation a try.

In a letter to a fellow doctor about his experience, Nettleton wrote:

Having too often found with no small Grief and Trouble, how little Assistance of Art cou'd avail in many Cases of the *Small Pox*, I was induced to try the Method of Incision or Inoculation which came so well recommended by several Physicians from *Turkey* and which had also been lately practised in *London*. This I thought sufficient to justify the Attempt.

Among the first patients he had in 1721 were the children of a Halifax family called Symons. He recalled:

There were four children, none of whom had had the small pox. I was called to the eldest who was seized in the natural way with the most malignant sort I ever saw, attended with the worst symptoms that could be, insomuch that he died on the fourth day all full of purple and livid spots. The parents were very desirous that any means might be used to preserve the rest; but here I was in great doubt and perplexity what part to act. I knew very well, that if I should venture to make an incision whatever should happen would be charged upon that, and it was not improbable but some of them might have already taken the infection.

It was a tough decision: if he inoculated and another child was already infected, their death, if it came, could be blamed on him. 'On the other hand,' he reasoned 'if it was omitted I did very much fear they might all dye [*sic*] such instances having been known and the contagion which was got amongst them being of such a destructive nature. Wherefore I was willing to run the risque [*sic*] of my reputation rather than that the children should perish.'[5]

Nettleton inoculated the three surviving children the day before their brother died, telling the parents there was no way he could predict how successful he would be. He would know if any of the children had already got smallpox if symptoms appeared before seven days after the inoculation. Tragically, one of the girls showed signs of infection on the second day and this was not at the site of Nettleton's incisions. She had full-blown natural smallpox the same as her brother. The girl survived a little longer than him, but died seven days after the inoculation.

The other two children 'got very easily through the Distemper'. The two children who died were infected before Nettleton's attempt to inoculate, but he knew very well that detractors would say he was responsible.

Between December 1721 and April the following year, Nettleton inoculated forty patients in the area of Halifax, most of them children. He was impressed and relieved by his success: just one patient could be judged to have died from the effects of inoculation. However, he proceeded cautiously, experimenting all the time regarding the best practice: deep or shallow incisions, and with a variety of potions to alleviate symptoms. Whatever method he used, he found that the results exceeded his expectations. The side effects of the children and adults Nettleton inoculated varied widely, some having very little discomfort and few pustules, others becoming quite ill before they recovered. Aware that what he was doing would be closely scrutinised in his home town,

Nettleton was relieved to be able to report that all but one of those he inoculated had recovered. One death in forty inoculations, if that was the true figure, would be regarded as catastrophic today, but in the 1720s it was counted a huge success. He wrote that he might have inoculated more had he 'pressed it' but he 'only took such as desired it for themselves, being cautious of perswading [*sic*] any Body to it, because I had but little Authority thereabouts to support me'.

So impressed was Nettleton's friend with the account he gave of his pioneer practice of inoculation that he sent it to the Royal Society, which judged it worthy of publication in its journal, *Philosophical Transactions*. There, it caught the attention of the newly appointed secretary to the Royal Society, Dr James Jurin. It gave him the idea of collecting statistics on the number of inoculations that had been performed, along with any records of resulting fatalities. The hazard, as he put it, of inoculation could then be compared with the hazard of risking an attack of smallpox in 'the natural way'.

Jurin was well qualified to conduct this research as he had graduated as a mathematician at Trinity College Cambridge and, after years as a school headmaster, had returned to Cambridge to study medicine. He was just 37 years old when he was appointed secretary to the Royal Society and took charge of its publications. Though he insisted he was open-minded about the benefits of inoculation, he was quite evidently in favour.

Before he could present a convincing case for the practice, he needed to discover how many inoculations had been carried out and what the fatality rate might be. To this end, Jurin put an advertisement in the Society's *Philosophical Transactions*, inviting all inoculators to contact him. By the end of 1722 he found that there had been precious few: just 182 performed by 15 different individuals.

Nettleton was top of the list with 61, followed closely by Dr Maitland with 57 – he had been in demand after the Newgate experiment and the inoculation of Lady Mary Wortley Montagu's daughter. The third most prolific inoculator was the Sergeant Surgeon to the King, Claudius Amyand, with 17. In Chichester, Sussex, a surgeon and apothecary working together had carried out 13 between them. Then there was a 'Woman in Leicester' who had a tally of 8, followed by those who inoculated 6 or fewer. Only 2 deaths, possibly as a result of an inoculation were reported: that is, 2 out of 182 or 1 in every 91 inoculations.

Jurin was sent further evidence of the success of inoculation from the other side of the Atlantic, where the preacher Cotton Mather in Boston, New England, had persuaded a doctor to trial inoculation in the teeth of opposition from the church and community. Mather had seen the Royal Society reports from Turkey and had also learned from his black slave that inoculation was common in Africa. At Cotton Mather's behest, Dr Zabediel Boylston performed 300 inoculations, the great majority of which were successful. There were 5 possible deaths, which gave a mortality rate of 1 in 60. This was confirmation that inoculation was not infallible, but that casualties were rare.

In today's world, a fatality rate of 1 in 60 for immunisation would be regarded as shocking, but in the eighteenth century it was so far below the mortality rate for the victims of smallpox caught in the natural way that, statistically at least, the risk was worth taking. Jurin did the best he could, with what scattered evidence there was, to calculate the expected mortality rate in a smallpox epidemic. Nettleton provided some telling figures from Yorkshire towns and villages, collecting what evidence he could in the winter of 1722. He wrote to Jurin: 'I have taken an account in this town, and some part of the country, and have procured the same from several other towns hereabouts, where the small pox has been epidemical this last year, with as much exactness as was possible, how many have had smallpox, and how many out of the number have died.'[6]

He set out the results in a table. The mortality rate due to smallpox was mostly around 20 to 25 per cent: in Leeds, of the 792 people said to have had smallpox, 189 had died. In Halifax, 43 out of 276 people afflicted were dead; 37 out of 302 in Macclesfield. Overall, out of the 3,405 smallpox sufferers from the towns and villages around Halifax, 636 had died, more than 18 per cent.

Nettleton commented:

I am very sensible you will require a great number of Observations before you can draw any certain conclusions. I would only crave leave to remark that it appears from these accounts, that this last year in this part of the Kingdom, almost nineteen of every hundred, or *near one fifth of those who have had the natural smallpox, have died: whereas out of sixty one which have been inoculated hereabouts, not one has died*

Jurin continued to appeal for estimates of smallpox mortality and was sent reports from Chichester in Sussex where, out of 994 people who were infected, 168 died, and from Haverford West in Wales, where, out of 227 infected, 52 died. Cotton Mather reported from Boston, New England, that, over six months, 5,000 people had been infected with smallpox of whom about 900 had died.[7]

Jurin was unequivocal in his judgement that inoculation was much safer than risking an attack of 'natural' smallpox. Of all children born, he thought about 1 in 14 would die of smallpox, whereas among people of all ages, 1 in 5 or 6 of those infected would die. Of those inoculated, perhaps 1 in 60 would die, although there was some evidence that the mortality rate was much lower. The experience in Turkey, where inoculation had been practised for a great many years, was that the fatality rate from engrafting was close to zero.

Despite the overwhelming evidence of the success of inoculation as a practice, it went into decline. Nettleton reported fewer inoculations after two years. He knew what he was up against from the start, stating in the first account of his experience:

> There is only one thing I am obliged to mention which I wou'd rather have pass'd over in silence, and that is the vigorous opposition it has met with from many honest well meaning persons, who cou'd not but fancy, that it is an unlawful and unwarrantable practice. I only wish that as they act upon a principle of conscience, they would have been less busy in raising or spreading false and groundless reports whereby this matter has been very much misrepresented, and, many, entertaining a wrong notion of it, have been deterred from making use of this method for themselves or their children, who have since been unhappily taken off by the *Small Pox*.[8]

Plus ça change!

4

A Rural Revolution

Though the part Thomas Nettleton played in the adoption of inoculation in Britain was brief, his pioneering efforts to find the best procedure, noble though they were, had an unfortunate consequence. Medical theories of the day held that smallpox originated in the body and that the pustules on the sufferer's skin were caused by an internal eruption. It followed that the incision in the arm or leg of the patient was to 'let the poison out' rather than introduce it through the skin.

Nettleton wrote:

> It is not material in raising the distemper, whether the incisions be large or small: but I commonly found, that when they were made pretty large, the quantity of matter discharged afterwards at those places was greater; and the more plentiful the discharge the more easy the rest of the symptoms generally are, and they are also by this means best secured from any inconvenience, which might follow, after the pox are gone off.[1]

As Lady Mary Wortley Montagu was at pains to point out, the successful method of inoculation she had witnessed in Turkey required only a pin prick to introduce the infective matter. But Nettleton, like other doctors in Britain, regarded this as a crude 'folk' practice which needed to be improved upon. A deep cut was more consistent with conventional medical wisdom.

In his *History of Smallpox*, written in 1815, James Carrick Moore said of Nettleton:

This physician, unfortunately was imbued with the old notion of humours; and he attributed much of his success to this peculiar method of operating. Instead of small punctures, he made an incision through the skin; near an inch in length, in one arm, and in the opposite leg: bits of cotton, charged with variolous pus, were then introduced into the wounds, and confined by plasters and rollers. The Doctor boasted of procuring by those means a plentiful discharge: he in fact excited two foul ulcers, which were considered of great utility; and obviated a theoretical objection which had been made to inoculation, that the peccant matter [virus] was not sufficiently evacuated. This plan was adopted generally and even Mr Maitland was driven from the Byzantine method of making slight punctures, to this more cruel and mischievous operation.[2]

In retrospect, Nettleton's method was not as brutal as that developed by those few doctors who chose to practise inoculation in the years that followed. We have no record of the various approaches that were tried but there is enough evidence to indicate that deep incisions were the rule and that the patient had to be 'prepared' in a very drawn out and tiresome fashion. It was all to do with getting the blood 'right', though it was never clear what that meant.

What it entailed was blood letting and purging over several weeks with a very restricted diet before the inoculation took place. Thereafter the patient was kept in a warm room until the disease had run its course. After eight weeks they would be able to breathe fresh air again. It was not a regime that many could afford in lost time or money. The wealthy would employ both a physician to administer medication and a surgeon to perform the inoculation. Servants who had survived smallpox and were therefore immune might be employed to care for children while the induced infection ran its course.

Others who were not wealthy enough for such luxuries could have a very unpleasant experience. Although he left no written account of it himself, Edward Jenner, celebrated later for his discovery of vaccination, was inoculated some time in 1756 or 1757 when he was 8 years old. It was a traumatic experience described in *Biographical Anecdotes of Dr Jenner* by a friend of his, Thomas Dudley Fosbroke, who called his treatment barbaric.

At a very early period of the life of Dr Jenner the foundation was probably laid for his subsequent investigations as to the Preventive of Small-Pox, by the following circumstances. He was a fine ruddy boy, and at eight years of age was, with many others, put under a preparatory process of Inoculation with the Small-Pox by the late Mr Holbrow of Wotton Underedge. This preparation lasted six weeks. He was bled, to ascertain whether his blood was fine; was purged repeatedly, till he became emaciated and feeble; was kept on a very low diet, small in quantity, and dosed with a diet-drink to sweeten the blood.

After this barbarism of human-veterinary practice he was removed to one of the usual inoculation stables, and haltered up with others in a terrible state of disease, although none died. By good fortune the doctor escaped with a mild exhibition of the disease. After this he went to Cirencester, to a school, at which he stayed a year; and upon his return home, at the expiration of the term, he had arrived at the end of the Latin Accidence. His health not being quite reinstated, he was consigned to the tuition of the Rev Mr Clissold at Wotton

Underedge; and at the same time put under the care of the eminent physician, the late Dr Capell. The effect of the preparation and inoculation just mentioned was this – as a child, he could never enjoy sleep, and was constantly haunted by imaginary noises; and a sensibility too acutely alive of these and sudden jars has ever since subsisted.[3]

Had Jenner been born not in 1749 but a few years later, he might well have been spared this ordeal, for it was not long before a revolution was under way in the favoured technique of inoculation, which was adopted all over the country. It was associated everywhere with the name Sutton. In fact, Fosbroke remarked how different Jenner's boyhood treatment would have been under Sutton's care.

It is not easy to appreciate now how it might be possible for a 'medical revolution' to take place when it involved absolutely no advance in the understanding of infections, nor any close studies of the effectiveness of different drugs or medical procedures. But 'Suttonian inoculation', as it came to be known, was a genuine breakthrough, and was recognised as such at the time by most medical authorities. It evolved from a rejection of customary medical practice and a partial return to the simplicity of the Turkish method of inoculation. Lady Mary's anecdotal accounts of the work of the elderly Greek ladies were probably more influential than any theories about the nature of disease. It was a rustic kind of revolution which began in the Suffolk village of Kenton in the mid-eighteenth century.

Very few country surgeons had attempted to inoculate before 1750. When they did they were routinely hounded out by the clergy and hostile townspeople. When, in 1742, John Rodbard, a surgical apprentice in Woodbridge Suffolk, experimented by inoculating himself, he was taking a bold step towards setting up a practice. There is no record of how he developed his technique, but it is likely that Nettleton's example was influential.

Whatever technique he had devised, Rodbard claimed in newspaper advertisements that his inoculations were always successful: no deaths and nobody seriously ill. It was a boast that came back to haunt him. In 1756 Rodbard was asked to inoculate the eldest son of another Suffolk surgeon, Robert Sutton. The two men knew each other and were apparently on good terms. Sutton was then nearly fifty years old and, in thirty years practising as a surgeon, had never attempted inoculation himself. Perhaps he was keen to see how it was done. His eldest son, also Robert, was no infant, but a strapping 24-year-old and the expectation was that he would recover without much discomfort from Rodbard's supposedly expert treatment. However, to the horror of his parents and his large family – six brothers and two sisters – Robert suffered a severe attack of smallpox which he was lucky to survive.

This traumatic episode in the life of the Suttons was the inspiration for the innovations which, in time, made their name synonymous with the safest and most successful practice of inoculation in the eighteenth century. Robert's younger brother, Daniel, was particularly affected and, years later, when he had superseded his father in reputation, he recalled with bitterness Rodbard's claim in newspaper advertisements that he had taught the Suttons how to inoculate. He published in the local newspaper a bitter riposte to the idea that Rodbard was their mentor:

Mr Sutton presents his final *most respected compliments* to Mr Rodbard; and as he has the *Modesty* still to insinuate that he first taught Mr Sutton's family the Art of Inoculation, he asks him if he remembers a little conversation that once passed between his father and him, in the company of an eminent Physician of Ipswich? . . . The following will refresh Mr Rodbard's memory. Mr Sutton's father was saying that he proposed to practise inoculation! What you! (exclaimed Mr Rodbard with his usual *sneering politeness*) I suppose you know much about inoculation. Yes, replied Mr Sutton, I know as much about it as you did when you began. Here the acquaintance ended, and Mr Rodbard from this Time commenced Enemy to Mr Sutton.[4]

Robert Sutton, the father, wrote nothing of this episode, in fact nothing at all ever, confining himself to advertisements in newspapers extolling his success with inoculation and hinting at his discovery of 'new methods' and special potions. However, later in life he had an unofficial biographer in Robert Houlton Jnr, a great champion of the Suttons and their methods. According to Houlton: 'Mr Sutton was so much concerned and tortured, as it were, for a while, for the fate of his son, and the extreme danger to which he had exposed him, had such an effect on his mind, that he determined, from the moment of his recovery, to dedicate his thoughts solely to the smallpox.'[5]

There followed, Houlton tells us, several months of 'study and consideration' before Sutton had the nerve to try out the scheme he had devised. Unfortunately, we learn nothing about what he was studying and little about what his considerations were. This can only be inferred from his subsequent advertisements. However, after one or two trials (one of them possibly on his son Daniel, who says he was inoculated in 1757), he went into business.

Robert Sutton's first-ever advertisement, published in April 1757 in the *Ipswich Journal*, revealed that he really had given great consideration to his new venture as specialist inoculator. Comfort and assurance were the keys to his sales pitch rather than any claims to originality in his method. He had hired 'a large and commodious house' for the reception of people who were to be inoculated by him. The terms were:

Gentlemen and Ladies will be prepared, inoculated, boarded and nursed and allowed tea, wine, fish and fowl at seven guineas each, for one month, Farmers at five pounds, to be allowed tea, veal, mutton, lamb etc. And for the benefit of the meaner sort, he will take them at three guineas for a month, if they are not fit to be discharged sooner; and those that can board and nurse themselves, he will inoculate them for half a guinea each.[6]

Sutton's practice grew from its small beginnings at a pace he could not have anticipated. By October he had two 'commodious houses' for his patients and the following year had built an entirely new house, while on market days he was available in several towns in Suffolk.

In his first year as an inoculator Robert Sutton had forty-one patients. The following year just twenty-seven. Then his fortunes rose as he gained a reputation, the numbers of his patients rising and falling year by year, fluctuations in demand almost certainly following the onset and disappearance of outbreaks of smallpox. By 1767, Robert Sutton and sons had inoculated 2,514 patients. His most prolific single year was 1763 with 575, by which time his eldest son Robert was practising on his own account in the town of Bury St Edmunds, and his second son, Daniel, after time away as an assistant to an apothecary, had joined him in the enterprise carrying out many inoculations himself.

It was at this time that Robert Sutton chose to reveal something of his methods of inoculation in advertisements in the *Ipswich Journal*. He claimed that in a few months he had inoculated 200 patients who had not on average more than 100 pustules each. Some of these patients were over 40 years old and had 'drunk very hard for fifteen or twenty years'. The slight reaction to his inoculations was a result of his 'new method' of inoculating, as he put it, 'without incision'. He claimed: 'the most curious eye cannot discern where the operation is performed for the first forty-eight hours.'[7]

Robert and four other of Sutton's younger sons were all happy, in time, to join their father's business and to promote his revolutionary approach to inoculation all over the country. They began to create a franchise whereby surgeons and apothecaries who wanted to adopt the Sutton method would pay a fee for the privilege. They could then advertise that they were properly trained. It was worth paying the fee if it brought in more patients. Inoculation was becoming a lucrative trade.

Robert Sutton had established a family business and had had his bumper year when his second son Daniel, now 28 years old, decided he wanted to set up on his own. He believed he could do better than his father by offering inoculation which would be more amenable to the patient. Legend has it that there was a fierce argument between father and son, but neither ever revealed publicly what took place.

Writing many years later, William Woodville, author of *A History of the Inoculation of Smallpox in Great Britain*, said he had known Daniel, who gave him an account of the reason for the rift:

in the year 1763 (he) suggested to his father (as I was informed by him) a new plan of inoculation, in which he proposed to shorten the time of preparation to a few days and not confine the inoculated patients to the house, but to oblige them to be in the open air as much as possible during the whole progress of the distemper. To reduce the process preparatory to inoculation from a month, which was then the usual time, to eight or ten days, was to obviate the objections that many persons had made to inoculation from the great length of time that it required.

This, therefore, might be thought a measure of expediency, to bring a greater number of patients; but obliging those under inoculation to walk out in the cold air during the eruptive fever, seems to have been a practice he probably discovered by experience. However

Mr Sutton, the father, could not be persuaded to adopt any innovation in the practice of inoculation and would not hear the whole of his son's new scheme, which he condemned as not only rash and absurd, but as extremely dangerous.[8]

Daniel left his father's lucrative business to seek his fortune with his new method of 'Suttonian' inoculation. He was brimming with confidence and determination. Inoculation against smallpox was still a novel specialism for a country surgeon and Daniel had no qualification. His father had been apprenticed, and took on apprentices, but Daniel was not one of them. He had just picked up the tricks of the trade from his father and knew that, given a chance, he could demonstrate his skills and make a fortune. As one those who employed him early in his practice wrote, Daniel Sutton was 'a most surprising fellow and hath a most amazing secret in giving and abating yer acrimony & venom of ye small pox'.[9]

5

A Most Surprising Fellow

In just four years, from late in 1763 until 1767, Daniel Sutton made a fortune working single-handedly as an inoculator. He did not, as might have been expected, head to London to prosper among the well-to-do. As he had no medical qualification it might have been risky. And in any case, his experience working with his father had taught him that in country towns and villages there was a demand for inoculation and not many country surgeons at that time were willing to offer it.

The village of Ingatestone in Essex that Daniel Sutton chose for his pioneer practice might look out of the way today, but in the eighteenth century it was a bustling stop-over en route from London to Colchester and the port of Harwich. This was the Great East Road, which was thronged with wagons and carriages, many heading for Harwich on their way to board the boats which regularly plied the southern North Sea to Holland. The Harwich route was favoured in 1763, when Daniel arrived in Ingatestone, for war with France had made the Channel crossing dangerous.

Travellers broke their journey at the inns that lined the main road through Ingatestone to change horses and spend the night. An advertisement for the sale of a lease on the Ipswich Arms and Chequers Inn in Ingatestone described it as 'one of the capital roads in the Kingdom for Coaches, Post Chaises and Drovers with pasture land, stables and a Barn'.

Daniel hoped to attract a new kind of clientele to the village, those who would come and stay at the inoculation houses he established just a short distance from the main road. They could not pop in for a quick jab in the arm. On offer was the same kind of treatment that his father had established, with patients living in the inoculation house for up to a month. To make his practice more attractive he would cut the time taken for inoculation and provide accommodation in a new and much more amenable way than was the common practice at the time. His patients would not be confined indoors, but encouraged enjoy fresh air while the pox developed.

Daniel was not known in the area and was aware that he would need some vigorous promotion to get established. This he did, as James Carrick Moore put it in his *History of Smallpox* 'with the old trick of puffing hand bills and boasting advertisements'. He began his campaign on 5 November 1763 with an advertisement in the *Ipswich Journal*:

This is to inform the publick [*sic*]

That DANIEL SUTTON, surgeon, has hired two very commodious houses in the parish of Ingatestone, Essex; in one of which (that
stands retired, and near two miles from the town), he proposes
receiving such persons as chuse to be inoculated by him for the
SMALL-POX. They are fitted up in a very neat and elegant manner,
and will be ready for the reception of patients the beginning of next
month.[1]

He tagged onto this first advertisement the one and only public acknowledgement he ever paid to his family: 'The extensive practice he has carried on with his Father at Kenton in Suffolk, for some years past, renders it unnecessary for him to mention their peculiar Method and great success. He hopes such favours from the public as his practice shall merit.' He must have believed the reputation of the Suttons was already established.

As luck would have it, a new newspaper, the *Chelmsford Chronicle*, began publication just as Daniel began his promotion. He was quick to add to the *Chronicle*'s column inches with a boast that attracted a good deal of attention. His patients could:

> quit their bed or room and take the air at any one stage of the distemper, except a few hours, whilst they are breeding it; having on average not more than twenty pustules each; a practice essentially interesting and worthy of the attention of the public, particularly the Fair Sex; as by this method the face is effectually prevented from being disfigured. By communicating the small-pox thus favourably, the patients in general are enabled to return to fresh company in three weeks, or less; a circumstance which particularly affects the working hand etc.[2]

By the end of his first year Sutton was raking it in. William Woodville reported in his *History of the Inoculation of Smallpox* that by the close of 1764, Sutton had earned 2,000 guineas: in today's money perhaps £400,000. The following year he more than tripled this income to 6,300 guineas and was well on his way to becoming a wealthy man. A local archivist, E.E. Wilde, in a history of Ingatestone published in 1913, wrote:

> seldom can a young man have earned so handsome an income by his own handi-work in so short a space of time . . . For those years our old road and village must have been thronged with pilgrims on their way to the new and fashionable cure, the coaches filled to overflowing, and inn-yards crammed with vehicles and beasts of all kinds, from the lord's smart chariot to the humble donkey of the cottager.[3]

This was not a trade popular with the local innkeepers and burghers however. No sooner had Daniel announced his arrival as an inoculator than the residents of Ingatestone were warned that he brought not prosperity, but danger and potential disaster. Adjoining one of his advertisements in the *Ipswich Journal* in November 1763 was an invitation to get out of town.

Information to the public

Whereas one Daniel Sutton has advertised that he has hired two houses in Ingatestone to inoculate the smallpox; this is to certify the public, that the neighbourhood of Ingatestone is at present entirely free from the smallpox and tho the said two Houses stand about one mile distant from the Town, yet they are close to a much frequented road and necessarily must have such a communication with Ingatestone that the infection must be spread in time if the project should go on, the principal inhabitants of this and the neighbouring parishes therefore are determined to give all the opposition thereto that the law will enable them to do; as infecting a Town of so much traffick will be to the detriment to the public, and may be easily proved a nuisance.[4]

This was quite a common reaction to news that a doctor was setting up as an inoculator in a town or village where there had been no smallpox for several years. There was no law against inoculation. Daniel knew that very well and was not at all perturbed. He responded with an advertisement saying there was no prohibition on the use he was making of his rented houses. He practised only as an inoculator and could not be threatened in the same way as country surgeons with a general practice, who might lose their standing in the community and their livelihood if they persisted in offering inoculation. The only time

Daniel came close to censure was once when, at the height of his fame in 1767, he faced a charge in the larger nearby town of Chelmsford that he had started an epidemic of smallpox by bringing in infected patients.

A grand jury, a kind of tribunal of the good and the great in the town, considered the charge and dismissed it for lack of evidence. He was not the only inoculator in town who might have started an epidemic and Sutton was sure that the charge was malicious, cooked up by his rivals. But the criticism continued, with critical coverage in the press, which now included the *Chelmsford Chronicle*. In May 1765, when Daniel was well established, an anonymous correspondent, probably an inn-keeper, posted a scaremongering piece that claimed that:

> many reports came to be spread about the country that are prejudicial to the interest of the inhabitants, by deterring travellers from stopping there. And whereas it has been said in particular that Mr Coverdale at the Swan had lett part of his house for the purpose of inoculation; This is to certify the public that no part of the said house has been let for that purpose and that none of Mr Sutton's patients have at any time to our knowledge laid in any of the inns of the said town during their state of infection.[5]

The proprietor of the Swan, the most prominent and popular inn, paid for his own advertisement in the *Ipswich Journal* of 6 July 1765 to dissociate himself from any of Sutton's activities, announcing that: 'For the future no letters or parcels whatever that shall be directed either to Mr Sutton or his patients Will be taken in at the Swan aforesaid; neither will he at any time Hereafter furnish the said Mr Sutton or any of his patients (during their stay with him) with any horses or chaises, upon any pretence whatever.'[6]

Banishment from the Swan Inn was water off a duck's back for Daniel. He was now established in Ingatestone with the wealth to buy a house called 'Maisonette' to which were attached 39 acres of land, the estate standing on a 'favourable' rise just outside the village, where it remains to this day. Daniel's income no longer came solely from his local practice but from a franchise system, which copied that begun by his father. Such was his growing fame that he had requests from doctors practising miles away in other counties to sign up as authorised Suttonian inoculators. There is no record of what they paid for the privilege, but it is likely that Daniel drove a hard bargain. When a doctor was signed up they would get an endorsement in the local paper, which served to enhance Daniel's reputation and promote the Sutton brand.

Not only were there Daniel Sutton acolytes everywhere, his father and four of his brothers were all advertising their special expertise so that in the 1760s, if there was a report by someone saying they had been treated by a Mr Sutton, there was no certainty as to which one it might refer. But whichever one it was, you could be certain that the routine was the same, involving as it did a meticulous attention to detail. At the same time, the inoculator would not be nervous or anxious but brimming with confidence. That was a Sutton hallmark.

Just two years after he broke away from his father's practice, Daniel had won for himself a reputation as *the* Suttonian inoculator. His rivals began to wonder what it was about his inoculation practice that was so appealing and, apparently, effective. One of those who engaged him was the Tory grandee and country gentleman, Bamber Gascoyne, a former lawyer and sometime Member of Parliament with a reputation for speaking his mind. Though he referred to Sutton as 'the pocky doctor' in letters to his friend John Strutt, Gascoyne was struck by Sutton's understated, but confident, professional manner.

He wrote to Strutt: 'My children I have seen today at ye farm and there met Mr Sutton who has been very punctual in his attendance, & if I may judge from what I have hitherto seen, is a most surprising fellow & hath a most amazing secret in giving and abating yer acrimony & venom of ye small pox.'[7]

Having hired Daniel Sutton to inoculate his three sons and a servant, Moor, Gascoyne was keen to observe the inoculator at work: as he wrote to Strutt: 'I will here give you an historical account to ye best of my observations that you may compare with other practitioners.' He believes Sutton's powders contain mercury, and another medicine administered to those under inoculation to be a preparation of antimony mixed with coral or 'some of ye testaceous powders'. In preparation, the children and Moor, the servant, were put on a strict diet. 'My children are pretty well considering they are starved. Moor looks as if he had slipd ye chains from a gibbet; and Tuesday next they will all be poxd, my fears I need not express to you who have so lately felt on ye same occasion.'

Sutton's method of inoculation was of special interest to Gascoyne, and held a surprise. The source of infected matter arrived in the form of a 'Mrs Wallis, wife to Joe Wallis late of ye Hundreds but now of Messing and with her daughter ... they were in ye chaise and the two ladies looked as well and were cheerful as if they were come upon a visit. He applied to my wife and self to point out which had the disease but this by looks was impossible, he might as well shewn us two young fellows and asked which was clapd.'

It was Mrs Wallis who was the one infected with smallpox:

She had about seven pustules with large white heads on them. The doctor thrust a lancet in one of them which he immediately applied to the arm of Bamber [his eldest son] and put so small a part of the ye point of ye lance under his skin that he was not sensible of ye points touching him. Then he put on his cloaths without plaister rag or any covering whatever and so practised upon the others among which was my tenant's ploughman . . . this man pursued his daily labours as usual . . . he was somewhat affected with chill, stupor and head ache on Fryday and on Saturday he had two pustules on his arm with high heads on ye top full of matter. On Saturday upon sight Sutton pronounced his having been ill and declared he would have no more and that they would sink and scale in three or four days which they accordingly have done and the fellow is perfectly well.

Although the Gascoyne boys and Moor, the servant, came to no harm from Sutton's inoculation, the experience was not painless for any of them. Gascoyne wrote to Strutt:

On Sunday Evening Moor at times was flushd in ye face & sickish; on Monday he was very sick, chilly, eyes painfull & headache in ye evening Bamber was affected in ye same manner vomited much but was always better for going out; Moor was too much cast down to stir & declared he was so feeble he could not support himself; on Tuesday he continued ye same, or rather worse & had a fever both nights as had Bamber & there appeared a few more red spots upon ye neck & arms.

Isaac fell next into ye same way on Tuesday morning & Benny perfectly cheerfull & merry; Moors Bambers & Isaac spots appeared with matter on ye edges of ye red & in ye midle. this day Moor & Bamber were free from sickness &c but had great pains in their arms Moor's arm was much putrified between ye pustles & very much inflamed; Isaac chearfull & down fell Benny, pale Cold Sick & Nose bleeding & so lethargic that he could not keep his head up or eyes open. Sutton came over ordered him to take ye air in ye fields Cold & a N East wind; however he recovered spirits upon this.

The final mark of success for the inoculations was the minimal number of pustules each patient had on them by the time they were taken off their starvation diet. 'The farming man goes to meat tomorrow and Moor & Bamber may eat butter and eggs to their pudding; Sutton declares them all out of danger and says they will not have 15 pustles a piece; he is to visit on Saturday and intends bringing physic for them.'

Gascoyne was impressed by the way Sutton's regime appeared to have tamed a fearful distemper. He wrote to Strutt: 'If this is ye small pox I would sooner have it than the ague.' And he contrasted the experience of the inoculation of his sons and servant with that of some of his neighbours who were treated by a different doctor. 'Mr Fanshaw's youngest daughter about three years old hath been inoculated by a Mr Lenhams has got well over but has been much peppered as has four other of his patients in this part of ye County, two of which are not yet able to walk for soreness on their feet although inoculated six weeks agowe.'

Though Daniel Sutton's exceptional gift of 'abating yer the acrimony & venom of ye smallpox' was widely acknowledged at the time he was practising, it might be protested today that he was a mere 'quack'. After all, he lived in the age of quackery, when the newspapers were full of advertisements for pills and powders for which magical powers were claimed. The *Oxford Journal*, in January 1766, offered 'Dr James's Powder for fevers, the smallpox, measles, pleurisies, quincies, acute rheumatisms, colds and *all inflammatory orders*, as well as those which are called, Nervous, Hypochondriac and Hysteric. Price 2s 6d the paper.'[8]

Sutton did claim to have 'physic' that helped alleviate the symptoms of inoculated smallpox. And he prepared his patients with a strict diet and some laxatives. But they were not bled and there was no suggestion that his special potions 'cured' smallpox. He managed the onset of the disease after inoculation with close observation, adjusting the regime to each individual. Some could return to a normal diet sooner than others. All were encouraged at some point to get out into the fresh air once the pox had appeared. This was the hallmark of Daniel Sutton's regime, the innovation which supposedly led to the rift with his father. Nobody, including Sutton himself, could say *why* his regime worked. But it was impossible to deny that his was the least dangerous, least unpleasant and most reliable approach to inoculation.

As it became more and more familiar, practised over a large part of the country by Sutton's approved agents, it had the effect of removing much of the fear that people had of inoculation. As James Carrick Moore remarked in his *History of Smallpox*: 'Daniel Sutton, with his secret nostrums, propagated inoculation more in half a dozen years than both the faculties of Medicine and Surgery . . . had been able to do in half a century.'[9]

Sutton was sometimes described as a quack because he had no medical qualifications. He was, in the terms of the day, a 'mere empiric'. But what he achieved with his regime was real, effective as a preventive against the most devastating disease of the age. He was more successful than his father and brothers because he made inoculation more accessible and less daunting with his relatively easy-going regime.

As inoculation had become more acceptable in the 1750s, there were occasional attempts to inoculate whole populations simultaneously to overcome the danger of the infection spreading to those who had not been treated. This provided a new line of business for Daniel. In 1766, he was asked to undertake an ambitious general inoculation in the Essex coastal town of Maldon. Like most towns, Maldon had not approved of inoculation and few procedures had been performed. A fierce epidemic of smallpox changed the minds of the town's burghers.

Those who had not had smallpox and were therefore not immune were identified and in a single day Daniel inoculated 487 of the townsfolk, the great majority poor, and ranging in age from an infant of one month to 80 years old. The trade of the town, which had been threatened with disaster, was revived and a notice put in the *Chelmsford Chronicle* in the summer to reassure visitors that Maldon was now free of smallpox.

There is no record of the charge Daniel made for his services, but it must surely have been a substantial sum (on occasion he advertised that he would inoculate the poor for 1 guinea). His reputation and his fortune made in a matter of just three years, the Great Inoculator sought to add some respectability to his fortune and to move up in the world. He was to become, in his pomp, a veritable Georgian parvenu.

6

Sutton the Parvenu

Greatly admired as he was for his skills as an inoculator, Daniel was aware that he was regarded socially as no more than an avaricious upstart. He belonged to no societies, medical or otherwise, he had no qualifications nor had he published anything more profound than a series of newspaper advertisements. Then, in the spring of 1766, at the age of thirty-two, with his fortune made, he began to take steps to enhance his status and reputation.

In just one year he hired a clergyman at the princely annual salary of 200 guineas to officiate at a small chapel he had built in Ingatestone for his pious patients. At the same time, he applied for a Sutton coat of arms, which would cost him a considerable sum in fees. While he maintained his home, Maisonette, in Ingatestone, he took up residence in a grand house in London. His social standing now assured, he married a rich young widow whose parents owned land in the West Indies.

While the chapel was under construction, Daniel placed an advertisement for a clergyman:

Inoculation is practised with such great success in Essex that Mr Sutton, of Ingatestone (who has already inoculated above ten thousand without losing a single patient) is going to erect a chapel for Divine Service to be performed on Wednesdays, Fridays and Sundays;

as many Gentry, his patients, have frequently hinted to him how agreeable it would be; and has engaged to give a clergyman that officiates the genteel salary of 200 guineas per annum.[1]

How many clergymen applied we do not know, but it was an enticing stipend, equalling the annual income of the most prosperous country vicars. The man Daniel hired was not, as might have been expected, a retiring character happy to care for the souls of the recently inoculated. Instead he made himself an avid exponent of the benefits of inoculation. He preached a sermon entitled 'The practice of inoculation justified', which must have been a comfort to his congregation, all of whom had chosen to be inoculated.

Revd Robert Houlton had no intention, however, of limiting his audience to the few souls in the chapel in Ingatestone. He had the sermon published 'neatly printed and stitched in marble paper', with some added notes and observations and a dedication to Mr Daniel Sutton, priced at 2 shillings. In part, Houlton's sermon was a convoluted case for regarding inoculation as consistent with the Christian faith (a view many churchmen would not accept) and in part a eulogy. First, he praised Lady Mary Wortley Montagu for her part in introducing the country to inoculation and then his paymaster for making a success of it in the teeth of opposition:

Many base methods have been contrived to obstruct you; but you have surmounted them all, and are now above the reach of prejudice and malice. You have the voice of the people, and above all the happiness to deserve it. These considerations and the respect paid to you by some of the first physicians in the kingdom should teach your contemptible snarlers to know your merit, and to know themselves.

Go on then, sir, and prosper. May your present unsullied success always attend you. May you live many, many years to do good. May your art be ever crowned with infinite recompense of reward to yourself and heirs; with joy and happiness to this nation in particular and to mankind in general.[2]

In an appendix to his pamphlet, Houlton writes that he has looked at Sutton's books and noted that he inoculated 1,629 patients in 1764, 4,347 in 1765 and 7,816 in 1766, a total of 13,792. In addition, his approved partners had inoculated about 6,000 more, so that in just three years there had been about 20,000 people treated by the Suttonian method.

With the Revd Houlton now handling his public relations, Daniel took the bold decision to set up his practice in London. In March 1767, he moved into a recently built mansion in Kensington, then on the rural fringes of London, which he named Sutton House. It stood roughly where the Albert Hall is today. There he found himself in elevated company. Anthony Butcher, a distant relative of Daniel, described the company he was now keeping:

The neighbouring property was Grove House, then the home of Anne Pitt, sister of the Earl of Chatham and aunt of William Pitt who, a few years later, would become Prime Minister. The south front of these houses overlooked about two acres of grounds, which sloped down to the market gardens of Brompton, with views of the distant Surrey hills. To the north was Kensington Palace, the grounds of which had been opened to the public at certain times since the reign of George I half a century earlier. A diary entry of Lady Mary Coke for 7 June 1767 notes 'the little Prince of Brunswick is inoculated by Sutton. The child, born the previous year, was a nephew of King George III.'[3]

It was the move to Sutton House which seemed to turn Daniel's head. That same spring he applied for a coat of arms. He later wrote 'it may thus possibly contribute to do away with the silly reports, either of ignorance or of some less honourable principle; and establish me on that due line and rank which I have ever wished to hold as a useful member of society'.[4]

Daniel must have spent some time with the heralds choosing a range of medieval iconography appropriate to his occupation. E.E. Wilde, in his *History of Ingatestone and the Great Essex Road*, was clearly amused by the local hero's pretension: 'That which was granted him could not have added to the pleasure with which his medical brethren regarded him, though it showed considerable sense of wit and humour in the designer.'[5]

Part of the citation conjured up by the College of Heralds read:

We . . . have in allusion to, and as a Memorial of his great Skill and unparalleled Success in Inoculation, devised, and do by these Presents grant and assign to the said Daniel Sutton the arms following, that is to say Argent, a Civic Crown proper, on a Chief Azure a Serpent nowed [twisted] Or and a Dove of the Field respecting each other; and for the crest on a Wreath of Colours a Demi-Figure the Emblem of Love holding the Hymeneal Torch All Proper with his motto TUTO, CELERITER, ET JUCUNDE.

The motto translates as 'Safely, quickly, and pleasantly'. The Greek physician Asclepiades coined it around 140 BC as a definition of how a physician should practise. As for the heraldry, Wilde discovered that Azure signified vigilance and perseverance and that the serpent was a symbol of Esculapius, the Roman god of medicine. In Sutton's coat of arms the serpent, suggesting wisdom, was pictured facing a dove, suggesting he was 'wise as a serpent, harmless as a dove'. He would have paid heralds several hundred pounds to concoct this ersatz accolade.

The grant of the coat of arms and family crest (his father Robert and his descendants were included in the citation) would have entitled him to have these emblems of superiority displayed on his carriage and for him to be addressed as Esquire. There is no record of whether or not he took advantage of this opportunity. Perhaps his new-found wealth made him anxious. In November 1766, before he moved in to Sutton House, he had been held up by a highwayman. A newspaper report said that on a Sunday night he had been returning to Leicester Street, Leicester Fields in London from Wandsworth, where he had been visiting a patient with smallpox, when he was stopped and robbed of his money in Vauxhall.

The grant of the coat of arms came through just four days before his marriage to a Mrs Westley, described in the *Ipswich Journal* as 'a lady whose Merit and Accomplishments are too great and apparent to need a Panegyrick'. Houlton was possibly the author of this item which read:

> Yesterday was married at Chertsey in Surrey by the Rev Mr Houlton, Author of the *Discourse in Defence of Inoculation*, the celebrated Mr Daniel Sutton, Surgeon, to Mrs Westley, daughter of Simeon Warlock of Antigua. Immediately after the Ceremony the new married couple set off for Sutton House in Gore, where a grand entertainment was given to numerous and polite company, and a Band of Music provided for the occasion.[6]

Mrs Westley was a young widow just 21 years old. In 1764, when she was 17, she had married a Somerset clothier. There was a brief mention in the *Bath Chronicle and Weekly Gazette* on 19 January: 'Last week was married at St James's Church in this city, William Westley, Esq of Shepton Mallet, to Miss Worlock, an amiable young lady from Antigua with a fortune of 4000l.[7] Her family were reputed to own most of the West Indian island of Antigua, which might explain the substantial fortune she had as a young woman. Her marriage, however, was brief: her husband William died barely six months after their wedding day at the age of thirty-four. There is no record of how and when Rachel met Daniel. It is quite possible that the Revd Houlton introduced them. He was a chaplain to the Earl of Ilchester, whose seat was barely 30 miles from Shepton Mallet.

With his wealthy young wife, his coat of arms, his mansion in fashionable Kensington and a thriving business, Daniel might have left the days of rejection and hostility behind. But it was not in his nature to rest on his laurels and he remained his combative self until near the end of his life. It is perhaps unfortunate that he had as his champions the Revd Houlton, and, by 1767 the clergyman's son, also Revd Houlton. Both became pamphleteers in Sutton's cause, the younger Houlton for a time a Suttonian inoculator himself. Of the two of them, Houlton Senior was the more strident.

In 1767, newspapers all over the country were strewn with classified advertisements for the Revd Houlton's sermon 'The practice of inoculation justified'. In the appendix on 'the present state of inoculation with Observations etc', Houlton lashed out in all directions. A Dr Baker who claimed to have studied Sutton's technique in fact knew nothing. An attempt the previous summer to blame Sutton for a serious outbreak of smallpox in Chelmsford was the result of 'groundless insinuations and misrepresentations.[8]

Houlton claimed that Sutton's success was partly due to 'an inestimable medicine by which he can prevent all danger and difficulty'. Reviewing the catalogue of claims and rejoinders in the appendix to the sermon, the *Monthly Review* remarked: 'We are friends of inoculation; wish well to Mr Sutton; but are sorry to see a *reverend son of the church* descend to the level of a mere *nostrum-puffer.*' Finally Houlton's florid style drew the dismissive: 'might not the chaplain to the Earl of Ilchester, easily be mistaken for the *merry Andrew* [i.e. clown] to some wonder working professor of the stage-itinerant.'[9]

A year after the publication of the Revd Houlton's sermon, his son weighed in with his own defence of Sutton. Robert Houlton Jnr graduated from Magdalen College, Oxford University before practising as an inoculator, having been instructed by one of the Suttons. He set himself up in Ireland, where there was still considerable opposition to the practice. His pamphlet, *Indisputable facts relative to the Suttonian art of inoculation* was published in Dublin in 1768, relating the history of the Sutton family and repeating much of the vitriol which his father had included in his Ingatestone sermon and appendix.[10] What notice the public and the medical profession took of this it is difficult to say. However, one useful piece of information Houlton Jnr compiled was a list of all the approved practitioners of Suttonian inoculation in the country and abroad.

Including the father, then in Norfolk, and six Sutton brothers in Paris, Oxford, the Isle of Wight, Yorkshire and two in London, there were fifty-seven surgeons and apothecaries who could, without censure from Daniel, advertise themselves as genuine Suttonian inoculators. A brother-in-law of Daniel, a Mr Hewitt practised with a partner in the Hague, there were ten Suttonians in Ireland, two in Wales, and in twenty counties in England from Dorset to Durham, and one each in the British colonies of Jamaica and Virginia. This was a very large territory to police, yet Daniel never ceased to berate any surgeon or apothecary who he thought was taking his name in vain.

A typical of example of one of these many ill-tempered exchanges broke out in the columns of the *Salisbury and Winchester Journal* in July 1767. A notice appeared headed 'Mess Suttons to the Public' warning that a Mr Duke, who appeared to be insinuating that he was in partnership with them, in fact had no connection to them at all.

> The happy and great success with which our practice has been long attended, has induced, from time to time, mercenary and envious men to strive to build a reputation on our Name, and to use every means, however base, to acquire a fortune by influencing the public in their favour ... we find it necessary to inform the Nobility and Gentry of the County of Hants and the City of Salisbury that no person has been instructed by any of our family ... except Mr Smith and son.[11]

In reply, Mr Duke posted his own notice in which he 'did not doubt' he could have become a partner of the Sutton family but to 'practise physic on such terms, as, I am informed, his partners do, is inconsistent with my notion of rational practice. I think it borders too much on quackery to purchase a name and medications of any man, without knowing what those medicines are, especially if the person of whom such purchase is made, should happen to be illiterate and ignorant of physic and surgery in general.'[12]

Illiterate and ignorant! Implying that Daniel Sutton was something of a charlatan. How could an ignoramus with no qualifications have any claim to medical expertise. Stung by this perpetual barracking Daniel issued a challenge published in various newspapers including the *Oxford Journal*: 'in order to shew how false such reports are, Mr Sutton offers a HUNDRED GUINEAS to any person who can prove he ever lost a single patient by inoculation – that any of his patients ever had Small Pox a second time – or that the constitution of any person was ever injured by his peculiar and successful method'.[13] There is no record of anyone claiming the prize, and the very notion of a self-styled surgeon offering a reward to anyone who can prove his claims are false must have been viewed with disdain by senior members of the medical profession. To challenge Daniel Sutton or to engage him in debate would have been beneath their dignity. On the other hand, it was not necessarily beneath their dignity to spy on him to discover what the secrets of his undoubted success were.

·⟨══════⟩·

7

Sutton's Thunder Stolen

Though Sutton had no medical or social pedigree, his success could not be denied. But it was never properly acknowledged by his rivals, who quietly went about the business of figuring out how he did it while sneering at his lowly origins. The eminent, fully qualified doctors who sought to discover Daniel Sutton's secrets rarely mentioned him or his family of inoculators by name. They were invariably referred to as 'a certain family', as if to identify them would be to bestow a dignity on them that they really did not deserve. After all, the Suttons probably had no idea themselves how they had more or less perfected the art of smallpox inoculation. There was no published theory nor any description. If you wanted to learn their secrets you had to buy them by becoming a partner.

Sir George Baker, a physician to the Royal Household, in his 'Inquiry into the merits of a method of inoculating the smallpox', published in 1766, wondered how a procedure which was discovered by accident could be so successful. He wrote: 'some of its most valuable improvements have been received from the hands of Ignorance and Barbarism.'[1] Sir George did not approach Daniel Sutton, but instead quizzed some of his elevated customers who had observed him at work. People like Bamber Gascoyne would have given a fair appraisal of how it was done.

For Sir George Baker it was all a bit baffling. Circumstantial evidence suggested that the incision with the lancet was minimal so that no blood was drawn, the medicines prescribed were not very different from those routinely administered at the time, the patients were not confined to a warm room after inoculation but were encouraged to go out into the open air in all seasons, and all meat and alcohol was prohibited until the symptoms had disappeared.

He concluded that the key was the 'cool' treatment, the innovation Daniel had introduced in the teeth of opposition from his father. He made the point that Dr Thomas Sydenham, a physician who practised in the seventeenth century, had first advocated this regime for treating fevers, so Sutton could claim no great merit there. And Sir George thought the very slight incision made by Sutton was not always effective. As for the medication, it did not appear to be anything more than a conventional prescription.

Some doctors went to work on Sutton's secret nostrums with a view to analysing the components. A London doctor, Thomas Ruston, had already concluded his research when he was presented with one of Sutton's 'secret nostrums'. He wrote:

> After the foregoing sheets of the edition were committed to the press, a very ingenious gentleman, who is well acquainted with Mr Sutton, and has been much conversant among his patients, brought me a quantity of the medicines which he uses in inoculating for the smallpox, and which were prepared by himself. They consist of a powder, a pill, and some drops; and in order that I might determine their nature and composition, I subjected them to . . . experiments.[2]

From his analysis he concluded that the chief ingredient was calomel.

If this was the magic drug that Daniel's father, Robert, had 'discovered' as a treatment during inoculation, it had a venerable history. It was an innocent-looking white powder prescribed for centuries for all manner of ailments. Its effect on an inoculation patient was as a purgative, a cleaning of the bowels. It killed parasites such as worms, if there were any. A tell-tale sign that it had been taken was often a mass of saliva in the mouth. The medical wisdom, well into the nineteenth century, was that calomel was beneficial because it purged the body of disease. In fact, calomel is a poisonous compound of mercury.

However, Dr Ruston was right: it played an important part in Suttonian inoculation, administered in small doses, the quantity dependent on the age and perceived health of the patient. But that could not be the secret of Sutton's success. There were too many other factors to take into consideration. What was needed was a large-scale comparative study of different approaches to inoculation to discover which, in practical terms, was likely to be most successful. But how to design such an experiment in the eighteenth century? There was only one answer: orphans.

In 1739 a Foundling Hospital had been established in London to provide care for the hundreds of children who had lost their parents or had been abandoned by them. From the day the first children were admitted in 1741, the hospital's policy was to have them inoculated. As more and more orphans were taken in, the inoculation was performed away from the hospital to avoid infection. All staff had to be immune either from inoculation or from a natural infection.

The technique used at the Foundling Hospital in the early days would have been old-fashioned. This changed when William Watson, a physician and scientist with a history of experimentation with electricity, took over responsibility for the well-being of the children in the hospital. He wrote in the introduction to his *Account of a Series of Experiments in Inoculation*:

The success of inoculation at the hospital has been such, as no practitioners need to be ashamed of. Very great success has likewise attended inoculation in many parts of this kingdom; even though it has of late descended into very illiberal hands. But among these last I do not mean to include a *certain family* [italics added], who have practised inoculation with great success.[3]

Watson was aware that there were many rival claims to 'best practice' and he wanted to discover as scientifically as possible which method was best, not only for the Foundling Hospital but for the wider public. Children were inoculated in a variety of infirmaries staffed by nurses who would play a crucial part in Watson's experiment. They collected the raw data which Watson used to assess the usefulness or otherwise of a particular medicine or choice of lymph.

Once the outbreak of smallpox on each child had run its course, the nurses counted the number of pustules that appeared anywhere on the children's bodies, except on the scalp: hair made it difficult to see them. This was no mean task as, in total, the 74 boys and girls inoculated in the experiments had a grand total of 2,353 pustules between them. If that appears shocking, Watson pointed that just a single person infected by the most virulent strain of smallpox might have an even greater number.

The regime they all followed was very much the same as in the Suttonian method: the children were given a meat-free diet for ten days before their inoculation. The incision was made with the tip of a lancet just nicking the skin. Watson wrote: 'No plaster was used on any of them as I had long since found it to answer no other purpose than to disguise the appearance of the punctures. As in a few of them, half a dozen perhaps, the punctures spread, and were sore about the time, or soon after maturation, a poultice of bread and milk answered effectually every purpose of outward application.' The children followed the 'regime' that

Daniel Sutton had popularised. 'When it did not rain, or the weather was otherwise unfit, they were out every day, during the whole process, in a field near the infirmary where they were inoculated, where nobody else resorted.'[4]

The children in Watson's trial were aged from six to twelve, boys and girls divided like so many sport's day teams into three groups. While all followed the same basic regime, Watson varied the medication and the source of inoculum with the idea of discovering which was most effective, as judged by the number of pustules recorded on the bodies of the children in each group. Within each group there were considerable variations, which demonstrated how differently patients reacted to exactly the same regime.

After a systematic study of how many pustules each of the boys and girls had in the different groups, Watson found little variation in the outcome: all the children, whatever variant of treatment they were given, did well. None died and none were seriously affected by the inoculation. Giving medication before and after inoculation, whether calomel or an alternative, appeared to make little difference. The source of the inoculum, whether the fresh poison Daniel Sutton favoured, or matter taken from a more mature lesion, did not seem to make a significant difference in the number of pustules children suffered. Children who took no preparatory medicine did not do much worse than the others.

Watson summed up his view of the best practice:

the most essential parts seem to be the insertion of ichorous [that is, watery] variolous matter by small puncture; a well regulated vegetable diet before and during the whole process of inoculation; and avoiding of heated rooms and heating liquors, particularly in the inflammatory state of the disease. These to me appear the principal points. The boasted effects of the medical nostrums of several inoculators, at however an extravagant price the possessors may rate them are, in my opinion, very little to be regarded.[5]

Daniel Sutton did not engage in any discussion with Watson about these findings and certainly did not change his established practice. His unofficial spokesperson, the Revd Houlton Jnr, in his pamphlet *Indisputable facts relative to the Suttonian art of inoculation*, noted: 'Dr Watson's plan is only to give an account of the success of inoculation in the Foundling Hospital in London . . . It cannot therefore be expected that a gentleman will speak very sanguinely in favour of a practice at a time when he is relating the success of his own.'[6] However, he recognised that Dr Watson had afforded the Suttons 'some respect'.

In fact, Watson endorsed inoculation as a life saver for everyone and paid a special compliment to the Suttons. 'I hold it as a truth, and I am not singular in my opinion, that inoculation, practised by any person whatever, in any manner yet devised, and at any time, carries with it, in general, less danger to the patient than the natural smallpox, under the direction of the most able and experienced physician. Whatever, therefore, can contribute to the perfection of this salutary practice, deserves the most serious enquiry.' Of the Suttons, the *certain family* referred to in his introduction, he wrote: 'They have deserved well; not only on account of some real improvements they have made in the process, but also for the confidence they have excited in the public, from which vast numbers have been inoculated, who otherwise would not.'[7]

This observation was not lost on Thomas Dimsdale, a surgeon in the town of Hertford barely 30 miles from Sutton's pioneer practice in Ingatestone. Dimsdale had been an occasional inoculator for a number of years and could not believe the stories he heard about a new method. It all seemed implausible, another quack boast. Fancy patients with just a few pustules enjoying fresh air and recovering with only a minimal amount of discomfort. Could this possibly be true?

For someone from Dr Thomas Dimsdale's background, whose grandfather and father were surgeons and who had studied at a hospital in London before setting up a practice in his home town of Hertford, where his family owned land, the notion that a mere 'empiric' might have discovered a revolutionary technique for inoculation was frankly astonishing. He was in his mid-fifties, a good deal older than Daniel Sutton, married for a second time to an heiress and the beneficiary of an inheritance from his own family.

Dimsdale did not need the income from his medical practice. In fact, he had given up his practice for a while and only contemplated a return to it as his family grew: seven boys and two girls, all but two of whom survived to adulthood. But then he heard about Sutton and was intrigued. He made enquiries, and found out what he could with the idea of perhaps borrowing this new method. No approach was made to Sutton himself or his family. Dimsdale could learn all he needed with a bit of sleuthing.

Which of Sutton's patients he quizzed is not known, but he would no doubt have been interested in testimony such as that of the Revd Richard Radcliffe, who had described his inoculation by a Sutton (it is not clear which of the family) in a letter to a friend which began: 'Inoculation has been practised in this country so much and with so great success, that it seems to have lost all its terrors. I am willing to flatter myself, that I was not presumptuous or confident upon the occasion; though certain it is, that I was never more happy and chearful [*sic*] in any part of my life.'[8]

That was a measure of how far inoculation had come from the days of Edward Jenner's 'veterinary experience'. The Revd Radcliffe *enjoyed* his inoculation experience and had such a slight attack he hardly knew he had been infected and had to be reassured that the smallpox had taken. Dimsdale recognised something had gone on which had made his own mode of inoculation obsolete, and he was determined not only to discover the key to it but to turn it into his own 'new method of inoculation'.

Dimsdale, Quaker though he was, appears to have been quite sanguine about his blatant plagiarism. In the preamble to the treatise he published in 1767, with the title *The Present Method of Inoculating for the Small-pox*, he sneered at the lowly empiric who had succeeded where he had not. 'I first heard, with the utmost satisfaction, that in some parts of the country a new and more successful method of inoculating was discovered, than had hitherto been practised. The relators gave incredible accounts of the success, which were the more marvelous, as the operators were chiefly such as by report could lay but little claim to medical erudition.'[9]

Astonished that an unqualified surgeon had made a breakthrough in the battle against smallpox, Dimsdale nobly determined to bring this great benefit to the public. Not a word about Sutton, of course. 'Knowing that improvements which would do honour to the most elevated human understandings are *sometimes fumbled upon by men of more confined abilities* [italics added]; and that in medicine, as well as in every other circumstance in life, it is our duty to avail ourselves as much as is possible of all discoveries tending to the common benefit.'

In a sense, Daniel Sutton only had himself to blame when Dimsdale's well-written and influential account of the 'new method' went into several editions and was in demand in several countries in Europe. When he first had success in Ingatestone, Sutton had put an advertisement in the newspapers to say he would be publishing an account of his methods. But this never appeared. He claimed later he wanted to wait until he had 'perfected his technique'. In truth, there is little doubt he wanted to keep his method secretive and lucrative, as it was saleable.

Sutton's spokesman, the Revd Robert Houlton Jnr, dismissed Dimsdale's claim to have discovered the secrets of the 'new method'. In his tract *Indisputable facts* he wrote: 'I am not disputing the safety of Dr Dimsdale's practice, nor that of any other man: all that I insist upon is that the Suttonian art of inoculation is singular, is confined to themselves and their partners, and cannot be attained by *report*. The externals of the practice are seen, but their fundamentals are hid.'[10]

The only way to prove the superiority of Sutton's method over all others, including Dimsdale's 'new method', would be a government-sponsored test. 'The subject is certainly of sufficient moment to deserve it. Were three or four hundred orphans appointed for the purpose, all cavilling would end . . . the superiority of the practice ascertained by comparison.'

The Revd Houlton's gauntlet lay unattended, while Dimsdale got on with making a name for himself with a method he summed up in his best-selling pamphlet:

Should it be asked then, to what particular circumstance the success is owing? I can only answer that though the whole process may have some share in it, in my opinion it consists chiefly in the method of inoculating with recent fluid matter, and in the management of the patients at the time of eruption. If these conjectures be true, perhaps we shall be found to have improved but little upon the judicious Sydenham's cool method of treating the disease, and the old Greek woman's method of inoculating with fluid matter carried warm in her servant's bosom.[11]

8

Sutton Misses the Boat

By 1766 Daniel Sutton had reached his zenith, apparently untroubled by the competition of Thomas Dimsdale and others who believed they had discovered the secrets of his success. It was then that Sutton learned that a whole new world of riches awaited him and his acolytes across the Channel. Smallpox was rife in Europe and Russia and yet inoculation was rarely practised and fiercely opposed where it was attempted. But news of the success of Suttonian inoculation, promoted indirectly by the translation of Dimsdale's guide to the 'modern method' attracted the attention of royalty, who were as vulnerable to the scourge of smallpox as their subjects.

England produced the most skilled inoculators and a demand for their services grew. Sutton's name would be top of the list and an early approach was made to him. In the autumn of 1776, Daniel had inoculated the children of the Prussian ambassador in London. An item in a number of newspapers in November stated that 'his excellency informed the King his Master of the extreme singularity, dispatch and safety of the practice. On this his Prussian Majesty sent a most gracious invitation and promised his protection and encouragement to any one of the Sutton family who would come and practice at Berlin.'

It might have been expected that the ambitious Sutton, still only 31 years old, would have taken the coach from Ingatestone along the

Great East Road to board a boat to take him to a whole new world of riches. But he showed no enthusiasm for such an adventure. The Prussian king had asked for 'any one of the Sutton family' and it was one of Daniel's brothers-in-law, a Mr Hewit, who travelled to Berlin. There is no record of how he got on, but he appears to have become established as an inoculator in Europe.

Shortly after the approach from the king of Prussia, a much more public appeal came from the great Empress Queen Maria Theresa in Austria. It was a tragedy in the Hapsburg court in Vienna which prompted the cry for help. In October 1767, her daughter Maria Josepha was due to marry Ferdinand IV of Naples and Sicily in Vienna. A great celebration was planned, and, waiting in the wings was Leopold Mozart who had gone to the Austrian capital in the hope that the court would commission a special piece composed by his 11-year-old son Wolfgang, already a celebrated musical prodigy. But there was to be no wedding. A smallpox epidemic struck, taking as one of the victims the bride-to-be.

Learning of the great strides being made in combating smallpox in England, the empress instructed her ambassador in London, Count Seilern, to ask King George's physicians if they would give an opinion 'in regard to Messrs Suttons Practice in inoculation'. After a month's deliberation they published their report in February 1768. A more mealy-mouthed assessment of the Suttons' contribution to the great improvements in inoculation could hardly be imagined. It began tentatively that they 'humbly beg leave to observe that no report whatsoever in respect of the *general* success of inoculation in this Country, can greatly exceed the truth; that for many years past scarce one in a thousand has failed under the inoculation of Small-pox *even before the time of the Suttons* [italics added], where patients have been properly prepared.'

'Messrs Sutton and others have communicated the small-pox with great success, and thrown some new lights upon the subject of inoculation, particularly with exposing patients to the open air ...' Of Daniel they wrote: 'It is said that Sutton has inoculated 40,000 patients *without losing one*. They are not able to ascertain the number he has inoculated, but believe that he has not always been successful, though he has failed so very seldom that they do not think it ought to be considered as any objection to his method.'

And then the final put down: 'The Suttons are undoubtedly in some respects improvers in the art of inoculation, but by applying their rules too generally, and by their not making proper allowance for the difference of constitutions, have frequently done harm. All their improvements have been adopted by other inoculators, and in the hands of these, the art seems to be carried to very great perfection.'[1]

We do not know if Daniel ever had a direct invitation to go to Vienna. Instead, the great adventure went to a Dutch inoculator who had learned the Suttonian technique in London. More requests for English inoculators came from some of the grandest monarchies of the eighteenth century, but Daniel never took up the opportunities which it must be assumed were open to him. In fact, there is only one record of him going abroad and that was some time later, when a brief newspaper report said that he had returned from the south of France.

Why did he miss the boat and leave others to reap the riches offered to inoculators overseas? How did he feel when Thomas Dimsdale and others enjoyed riches beyond Daniel's imagination with their copycat versions of his Suttonian technique? The fact that he never complained about it publicly suggests that he felt he could not cope socially with the rarefied world of royalty.

There is no doubt that Daniel was socially rough and ready. It was said that Dimsdale began to take from him the more refined patients, one of whom wrote 'the terms of Sutton are so moderate that men in mean circumstances, men of low education and dissolute life, repair to his house, which is so confused and disorderly a place that one would admire that one tenth part of his patients do not perish by their irregularities'.[2]

A glimpse of Sutton's gaucheness in polite society is recorded by eighteenth-century diarist Mrs Hester Lynch Thrale, one of whose children was inoculated by Daniel. She introduced the man she called 'the famous Daniel Sutton . . . who first reduced the practice of communicating the Smallpox almost to a Certainty' to her elevated social circle. Present was Dr Johnson, who proceeded to address the company on the subject of money. With characteristic wit, Johnson mused that money was like poison, because 'given in large doses . . . it might sometimes prove destructive to a weak constitution, yet it might be found to work itself off and leave the patient well.'

Mrs Thrale noted: 'Sutton listened and grinned and gaped and said at last – half out of breath *I never kept such company before and cannot tell how to set about leaving it now* – the compliment, though awkward, pleased our Doctor much and no wonder, it was likely to please both vanity and virtue.' She came to the conclusion that Sutton was 'a fellow of very quick Parts . . . though as ignorant as dirt both with regard to books and the world'.[3]

For whatever reason, Daniel did not go to Vienna. That would have been prize enough, as the fortune of the man who went in his place will attest. But an even greater opportunity arose at more or less the same time when an emissary from Catherine the Great, the Russian empress, arrived in London late in 1767 to seek an inoculator to go to St Petersburg. An outbreak of smallpox had claimed the life of a nobleman's daughter and Catherine feared for her son. *Town and Country Magazine* reported that the Russian ambassador, Count Mussin-Pushkin, had sent for a 'Doctor-S', but Sutton said he would not go to Russia unless he was given £4,000 in advance.[4] The Sutton family tradition later had it that he had turned down £2,000. But there is no evidence either way for these stories.

All we know is that Sutton did not go to Russia. What we do know is that Thomas Dimsdale was put forward to the Russian emissaries as an equally experienced inoculator.

He was not nearly as famous as Sutton: if fact he was still then a modest country surgeon who happened to author a successful pamphlet on 'the new method' of inoculation. It had been translated into Russian, but it is doubtful he was well known there. But it was most probably Sir John Pringle, a Scottish military surgeon, who gave him a recommendation. A champion of Suttonian inoculation, Sir John had met Dimsdale in 1745 when they were both engaged in the Duke of Cumberland's campaign to suppress the uprising of Scottish Highlanders.

Dimsdale first of all declined the invitation to go to St Petersburg. He had not the slightest intention of going abroad. He wrote later in *Tracts on Inoculation* in which he gave an account of his Russian adventure: 'I was happily in possession of a fortune equal to my wishes, engaged in a considerable and profitable employ, and the still more endearing attachment to a large family. All these were reasons for me to decline the offer.'[5] He was not an ambitious young man, as he pointed out, but 56 years old, with a wife and seven children.

However, a special envoy was sent directly from Catherine the Great's court in St Petersburg, making the journey to England in just sixteen days, which impressed Dimsdale. He was entreated, as he put it, to 'introduce inoculation to St Petersburg'. The urgency, he discovered, was the result of another tragic death in the aristocracy. Yet another tragedy of a young bride suffering a fatal attack of smallpox before her wedding day.

Finally, Dimsdale agreed to go and embarked on an adventure which would transform his life and his status in a way which put Daniel Sutton's fortune and fame in the shade. With a grant of £1,000 for travel expenses, accompanied by his son Nicholas who was studying medicine in

Edinburgh and was familiar with his father's method of inoculation, he set off in July for St Petersburg. The journey took only a month. They were given lavish quarters and fêted by noblemen.

He soon discovered, though it was supposed to be a secret, that he was not only to inoculate Catherine's son, but the empress herself. This was a huge and unexpected responsibility. He would need a safe and speedy passage out if anything went wrong. Catherine the Great, he discovered, despised Russian doctors just as much as Lady Mary Wortley Montagu had despised English ones in the 1720s. Inoculation was not unknown in Russia but, where it was practised, it had not undergone 'modernisation' as it had in England. The empress did not want any of her doctors involved and said they would be useless anyway, because they did not understand the principles or techniques of inoculation.

In medicine, as in other aspects of life in the Russian Empire, Catherine thought of herself as a moderniser. Her determination to introduce inoculation was motivated not only by a fear of more deaths in families of the nobility, but also her belief that if it were adopted on a wide scale it would reduce the death rate and increase Russia's population. She was greatly influenced in this by the French philosopher Voltaire, who argued that improved medicine, and inoculation in particular, increased the wealth of a nation. Catherine's own inoculation, provided it was successful, would be symbolic, a message to her subjects demonstrating the safety of the procedure.

Dimsdale had many meetings with the empress, going each day to her chamber and talking until she had to take care of other matters. They seemed to get on well though they knew little of each other's language. As was customary at the court, Catherine spoke French, but that was not much help to Dimsdale. In a letter home, a Scottish merchant, John Thomson, who was based in St Petersburg and knew something of Dimsdale's relationship with Catherine, wrote:

He spoke so bad French as not to be able to explain himself intelligibly and what she comprehended whet'd her desire to know all and comprehend what he said to reconcile her to the arduous undertaking she meant him to undertake . . . She made the doctor speak to her in English what she could not comprehend in French . . . She accustom'd herself to treat him like an old man and intimate friend . . . she was charmed with the simplicity of the doctor and determined to be inoculated.[6]

We can only imagine how she might have got on with Daniel Sutton. Even at this distance it seems a shame that he did not meet Catherine the Great. Had he been her inoculator he would not have needed his expensive coat of arms.

Before he announced he was ready to inoculate either the empress or her son, the grand duke, Dimsdale consulted their doctors to learn about their general health. Though the royal doctors agreed to help with information about the empress and her son, none wanted anything to do with the inoculation. The fear that it might go wrong was palpable. But the empress expressed absolute confidence in Dimsdale. The original plan had been to inoculate the grand duke first, but this was postponed because of his poor health.

After following a diet prescribed by Dimsdale for a week, very much the Suttonian abstinence from meat, liquor and so on, the empress was inoculated on the evening of 12 October at the palace in St Petersburg. The next day she travelled to one of her country palaces where she was to stay until she was clear of the infection. She did not have an easy time of it, her sickness, pains, discomforts and uneasy nights duly documented by Dimsdale in his account, written in the form of a diary. He does not say whether at any point he considered Catherine to be in danger, but it must have been a very anxious time. He observed the

Suttonian rule of encouraging the patient to enjoy fresh air when the fever took hold. It was not until 1 November that Catherine had recovered and was able to return to St Petersburg.

The grand duke was successfully inoculated the day after his mother returned to St Petersburg. Twenty days later, on 22 November, he was fully recovered and Dimsdale was able to announce that mother and son were in full health. Dimsdale wrote:

> Immediately after the recovery of the Grand Duke, a nobleman of the first distinction acquainted me with the honorable and generous manner in which her Majesty proposed to reward my services; and particularly that I should be created Baron of the Russian Empire, and appointed actual counselor of state and physician to her Imperial Majesty, with an annuity of five hundred pounds a year to be paid me in England; besides ten thousand pounds sterling, which I received immediately; and also that I should be presented with a miniature of the Empress and another of the Grand Duke, as a memorial of my services to the Imperial Crown of Russia.[7]

Dimsdale's 20-year-old son Nicholas was also made a baron and presented with a gold snuff box, 'richly set with diamonds'. They were both subsequently in demand by the St Petersburg nobility to inoculate themselves and their children and the Dimsdales did not return home for four months.

Meanwhile, in Vienna, smallpox inoculation had been successfully introduced by another exponent of the 'new method', not a paid-up Suttonian, but a medic who had been instructed in the art while working in London. The epidemic which had led to the appeal for help had nearly killed young Mozart and his sister. Their father, Leopold, who was so keen for his prodigy to compose a piece for the royal wedding that was cancelled, had refused to have his children inoculated. He had written: 'I leave the matter to the grace of God.'

As the epidemic took more and more lives, Leopold reluctantly left Vienna, but not before both Wolfgang and his sister, nicknamed Nannerl, fell ill. He was lucky that they recovered and that they were not badly scarred. However, there was shock: Wolfgang was blind for nine days before he recovered his sight. When he returned to Vienna, Leopold wrote to a friend: 'Do you know that inoculation for smallpox is proceeding steadily here? The Empress has engaged the English inoculator to perform near the Schönbrunn palace. Already forty poor children have been inoculated satisfactorily. The Emperor and Empress come to the centre almost daily and are completely won over by it.'[8]

Not unreasonably, Leopold had assumed that the inoculator who had answered the empress's call for help was English. In fact, he was a 48-year-old Dutch doctor and a one-time assistant to Watson at the Foundling Hospital. He knew Thomas Dimsdale as well and had assisted him as an inoculator in Hertford.

Born in 1730, Jan Ingen-Housz was the son of a prosperous leather merchant who also practised as a pharmacist. He was said to have excelled in classical languages at Breda Latin school and had no inclination to study medicine. It is probable that his mind was changed by the arrival in a village close to Breda of a detachment of British troops stationed there as allies of the Dutch in the so-called War of Austrian Succession.

The British physician-general accompanying the forces was the Scottish doctor John Pringle, who became a friend of Jan's family. Jan's interest turned to medicine, which he studied at universities in Holland. He established a medical practice back home in Breda, but abandoned it when his father died. His brother took over both the leather and the pharmacy businesses, leaving Jan with an inheritance which gave him the funds to study in Edinburgh and Paris.

With Pringle's patronage, Ingen-Housz met many of the leading scientists of the day, including Joseph Priestley and the American Benjamin Franklin, an inoculation enthusiast, who became a life-long friend. He soon learned of Daniel Sutton's revival of inoculation with his revolutionary procedure, and was introduced to William Watson at the London Foundling Hospital. In 1766, Watson took Ingen-Housz on as an inoculator. In time, Watson handed over much of his inoculation work at the hospital to Ingen-Housz and soon he had a thriving private practice as well. He was an admirer of Thomas Dimsdale, who he assisted in the inoculation of two whole villages in the bitter winter of 1768. Called out to tend to a boy whose life he could not save, and fearing for the survival of the village, Dimsdale offered to inoculate anyone who put themselves forward. He waived the fees and was asked to offer the same to a neighbouring village. Ingen-Housz came in to help him with this impromptu general inoculation.

Within months, Ingen-Housz had left the modest homes of Essex villagers behind for the splendours of Empress Maria Theresa's court. He was invited on the recommendation of Sir John Pringle, whom he knew from childhood, the same military surgeon who had put forward Dimsdale's name to Catherine the Great's emissary. When he arrived in Vienna, Ingen-Housz was first asked to operate on forty children from poor families who were paid a small amount for taking part. It was a re-run of the 1721 test inoculations in London in Newgate prison, and among the orphans of St James's. Ingen-Housz then proceeded to inoculate the empress herself and many others, after which he was appointed court physician and councillor and awarded a life-long pension of £40,000 a year.

While he was in Vienna, Ingen-Housz was elected a member of the Royal Society in London in his absence. Sir John Pringle and Dr William

Watson were two of his sponsors. He spent six years in Vienna, married there and then, and with his substantial pension, was able to concentrate on electrical experiments. Later, in collaboration with Joseph Priestley, he discovered the process of photosynthesis whereby plants convert sunlight into chemical energy. He dedicated his book *Experiments upon vegetables*, published in 1779, to Pringle, of whom he wrote 'no man upon earth can have stronger reasons for a due sense of gratitude than I acknowledge to you'. With the huge pension he was awarded in Vienna, Ingen-Housz was able to pursue his scientific studies without having to earn a living and he spent his last days in England conducting experiments on plant growth.

It was his knowledge of Suttonian inoculation that made Ingen-Housz's fortune. But that was nothing compared with the riches lavished on Thomas Dimsdale: his Russian adventure not only made him a good deal wealthier, it also raised his status when he returned to his practice in Hertford. His detractors thought him pompous as he insisted on being addressed as 'Baron Dimsdale' and signed himself as such. He became a banker and was elected as Member of Parliament for Hertford. The empress called him back to Russia to inoculate her two grandsons and he made the journey again. His second wife, Anne Iles, with whom he had had seven sons and two daughters, died in 1779, and it was his third wife Elizabeth who accompanied him on his return to Russia. His rich and exciting life came to an end in 1800 without him ever once crediting Daniel Sutton for a fair portion of his good fortune.

9

A Suttonian in America

In Britain, there weren't really any challenges to the Suttons' claim of their inoculation method's originality. Dimsdale simply copied their methods as far as he could deduce them without signing up as a partner. Ingen-Housz learned the basics from Watson at the Foundling Hospital. However, most of those who practised the new method in Britain were members of the Sutton family or practitioners who were credited, having bought the Sutton seal of approval.

Not many tried their luck abroad. In particular there seemed to be little incentive to set up in practice in the American colonies. Smallpox inoculation had been pioneered in Boston in 1721, the same year as the Newgate trial in London. In some of the thirteen counties of colonial America it had been banned altogether, in others it had been practised with considerable success. Why cross the Atlantic for such a unprom-ising venture?

One who did was James Latham, an army sergeant who, before he was posted to Quebec with the threat of revolution growing in the colonies to the south, had got himself accredited as a Suttonian inoculator. After a slow start he built up a practice, finally settling in New York, and made himself a fortune. However, he came to an unfortunate end. Caught up in the battle of loyalties between Patriots and Royalists he found himself the butt of wild accusations of quackery and plagiarism. Americans, he found, reckoned *they* had invented the Suttonian system of inoculation before the Suttons. It was the first and only time that Daniel Sutton's claim to originality had been seriously challenged. Which is perhaps not surprising, as Latham had laid claim to be the sole legitimate Suttonian inoculator in the whole of what was then British North America.

In 1767, on the eve of his posting to Quebec with his regiment, Latham had signed a contract with William Sutton, a younger brother of Daniel, which proclaimed:

Whereas, William Sutton of Kensington Lane, in the County of Surrey, in England, hath found out and discovered a method or art of inoculation for the smallpox ... in order to extend the benefit of this method to America, did take James Latham into partnership for the carrying on and practising of this said method, art or mystery ... aforesaid in certain districts in America, with power to depute under him other persons ... under certain terms and conditions.[1]

Latham's first venture in North America hardly reflected this grandiose ambition. His first patients were men in his regiment, who paid him a guinea for each inoculation. He then began to advertise in the *Quebec Gazette* and to establish a small private practice. When epidemic smallpox broke out in Montreal, he moved there and opened up an inoculation house.

Latham extended his influence, establishing a franchise arrangement with partners, which was a direct copy of Sutton's in England. He clearly imagined he would emulate Daniel Sutton's success of a decade earlier as he sold on the rights to use the Sutton name to American doctors prepared to pay the fee. A note by a doctor practising in New York outlined the draconian terms demanded by Latham:

1. Daniel Sutton, by an unknown artist in E.E. Wilde's *Ingatestone and the Essex Great Road with Fryerning.*

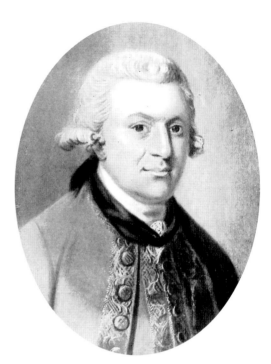

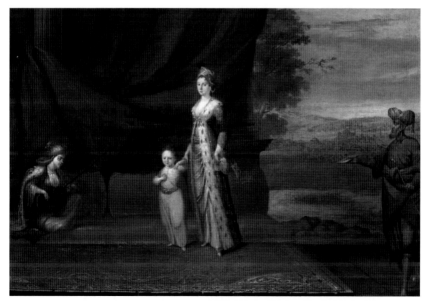

2. Lady Mary Wortley Montagu in Istanbul with her young son Edward, whom she had inoculated against smallpox in 1721 when in England it was considered a barbarous procedure which doctors refused to perform. Lady Mary's bravery began the acceptance of inoculation which later led to vaccination.

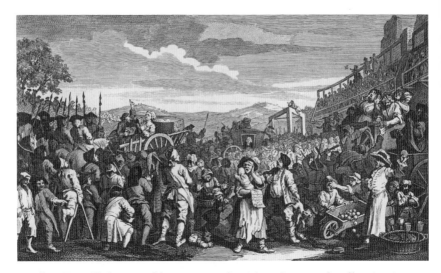

3. William Hogarth's depiction of the excitement of an eighteenth-century day of hangings in London, when the condemned went in procession from Newgate Prison to Tyburn. In 1721 six prisoners escaped this fate by volunteering to test the safety of inoculation against smallpox. The experiment was sponsored by royalty.

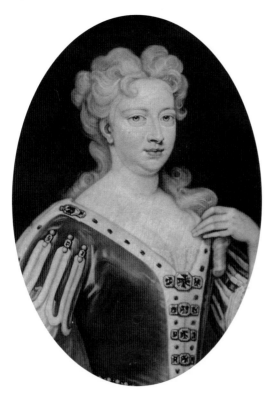

4. Princess Caroline of Ansbach had two of her daughters inoculated against smallpox when all the Newgate prisoners survived the procedure and some London orphans used as guinea pigs were paraded to demonstrate its safety. Eminent doctors were cautious but King George I gave it his blessing.

5. William Wagstaffe, a Fellow of the Royal College of Physicians, had witnessed the inoculation of the Newgate prisoners. He thought inoculation against smallpox was 'an experiment practiced by a few *Ignorant Women* amongst an illiterate and unthinking People . . . yet it was to be received into the *Royal Palace*'.

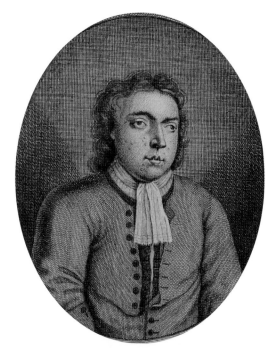

6. James Jurin, secretary to the Royal Society, collected evidence of the success of smallpox inoculation in saving lives, and produced the first statistics to show that it was safer than catching the virus 'in the natural way'. It took a long while for this to be accepted as fact.

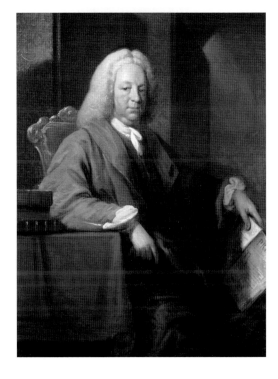

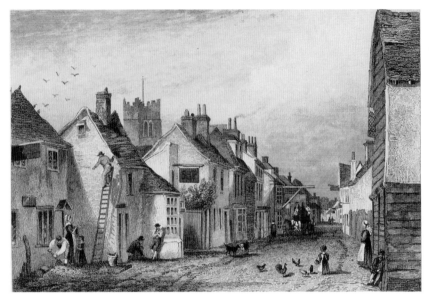

7. The high street in the Essex village of Ingatestone which straddled the main route between London and the busy port of Harwich. It was here in 1763 that Daniel Sutton began his revolutionary inoculation practice in the teeth of much fearful local opposition.

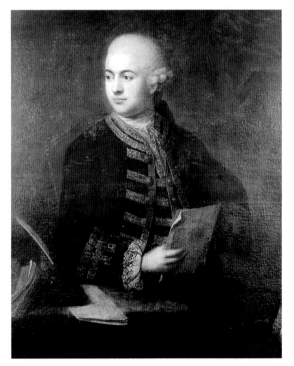

8. Daniel Sutton's family liked to claim that this portrait of him was painted by Sir Joshua Reynolds. Alas, the National Portrait Gallery can find no evidence for this. It captures Sutton at the height of his pomp when he bought himself a coat of arms and lived like a gentleman.

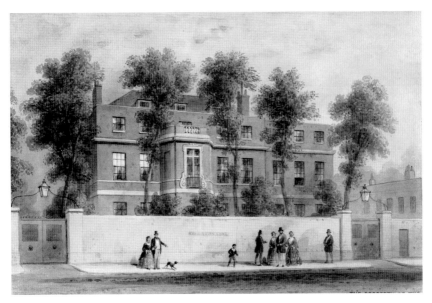

9. After his spectacular success inoculating in Ingatestone, Sutton moved up in the world acquiring a new property in the new suburb of Kensington. In Sutton House (later Grove House where the Albert Hall stands now) he rubbed shoulders with the aristocracy, but he was never accepted into London society.

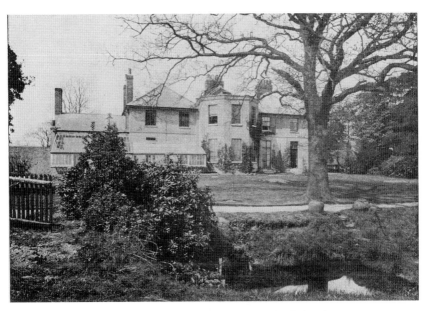

10. Sutton lived much of his life at different addresses in London but he kept his roots in Ingatestone with a house and estate he bought when he first made money. It was called Maisonette and stayed with his family long after his death. The house survives to this day.

LATELY PUBLISHED,

THE

PRESENT METHOD

OF

INOCULATING

FOR THE

SMALL-POX.

To which are added,

Some Experiments, inftituted with a View
to difcover the Effects of a fimilar Treatment in the NATURAL SMALL-POX.

By THOMAS DIMSDALE, M.D.

The SEVENTH EDITION, Corrected.

11. Sutton's thunder was stolen by Thomas Dimsdale, an older Essex surgeon, who saw the profits to be made from what he called 'the new method of inoculating the smallpox', and published an account of the technique he had learned from questioning Sutton's patients.

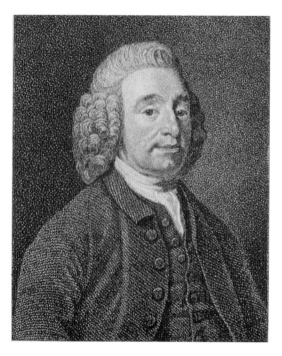

12. Thomas Dimsdale took on the risky commission to inoculate Catherine the Great of Russia. It was a huge success: he was given the title of baron, which he flaunted back in England, and became very wealthy. Though he stole Sutton's technique of inoculation Dimsdale never mentioned him by name.

13. In 1798 a country surgeon named Edward Jenner privately published an account of why he believed cowpox could protect against smallpox, providing a safe form of inoculation. Jenner named cowpox *variolae vaccinae*, meaning 'smallpox of the cow'. The adoption of vaccination was the beginning of the end for Sutton's fame.

AN

INQUIRY

INTO

THE CAUSES AND EFFECTS

OF

THE VARIOLÆ VACCINÆ,

A DISEASE

DISCOVERED IN SOME OF THE WESTERN COUNTIES OF ENGLAND,

PARTICULARLY

GLOUCESTERSHIRE,

AND KNOWN BY THE NAME OF

THE COW POX.

BY EDWARD JENNER, M. D. F. R. S. &c.

——— QUID NOBIS CERTIUS IPSIS
SENSIBUS ESSE POTEST, QUO VERA AC FALSA NOTEMUS.

LUCRETIUS.

London:

PRINTED, FOR THE AUTHOR,

BY SAMPSON LOW, N°. 7, BERWICK STREET, SOHO:

AND SOLD BY LAW, AVE-MARIA LANE; AND MURRAY AND HIGHLEY, FLEET STREET.

1798.

14. Edward Jenner became the great hero in the fight against smallpox. However, his notoriety waxed and waned. This statue by William Calder Marshall was unveiled in Trafalgar Square in 1858. Four years later the discoverer of vaccination was not thought distinguished enough for the honour and was moved to Kensington Gardens.

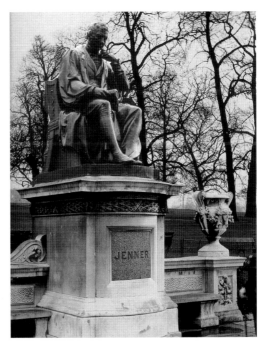

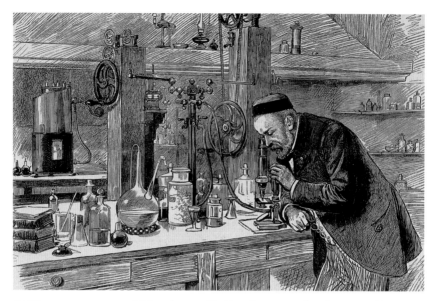

15. Microscopes more powerful than those used by Daniel Sutton or Edward Jenner enabled scientists to discover for the first time the microbes that caused disease. The French chemist and microbiologist Louis Pasteur (pictured) sealed Jenner's reputation by proposing that in his honour all inoculations against disease be called vaccines.

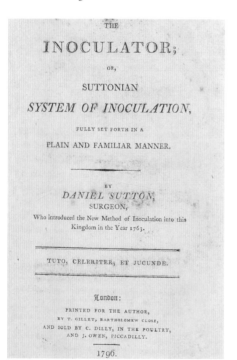

16. Sutton's one and only publication *The Inoculator* was considered obsolete almost as soon as it was printed in 1796. The secrets of his undoubted and remarkable success in combating smallpox were important for the development of vaccination which was regarded as a better form of Suttonian inoculation.

THE

INOCULATOR;

OR,

SUTTONIAN

SYSTEM OF INOCULATION,

FULLY SET FORTH IN A

PLAIN AND FAMILIAR MANNER.

BY

DANIEL SUTTON,
SURGEON,

Who introduced the New Method of Inoculation into this Kingdom in the Year 1763.

TUTO, CELERITER, ET JUCUNDE.

London:

PRINTED FOR THE AUTHOR,
BY T. GILLET, BARTHOLOMEW CLOSE,
AND SOLD BY C. DILLY, IN THE POULTRY,
AND J. OWEN, PICCADILLY.

1796.

The remedy was kept secret by the inventor, Dr William Sutton, of Surrey in England, except from those who purchased knowledge ... Dr Latham, surgeon in his majesty's 8th regiment of foot, partner and agent of Sutton ... licensed physicians to administer the medicines prepared and furnished by himself within certain towns and limits, they contracting to pay over to him one half of all monies received, until his portion should amount to three hundred pounds, and afterwards one third of all further sums obtained in the business; and covenanting not to attempt by analysis or otherwise, to discover the composition of the medicines.[2]

For a number of years Latham got away with this and began to amass a fortune as he moved from Quebec, to Montreal and then to New York, where he acquired a substantial property and farm. But, as revolutionary fervour gathered momentum after 1776, the claim that the 'Suttonian' method was superior to anything that was available in America eventually got him into serious trouble.

Latham had announced his arrival in New York in 1770 with an advertisement in the *New York Gazette and Weekly Advertiser* in which he boasted of the 1,250 patients he had inoculated in Quebec and Montreal.[3] He made a name for himself in New York with his 'Inoculation Apartments' on Broad Street. He had a chain of hospitals, five in the province of New York, and one at Worcester, Massachusetts. Latham advertised that 'any practitioner of character' might be accredited as a Suttonian inoculator by application. Classes were held in a number of hospitals.[4] He authorised a Dr Shuttleworth, a brother-in-law of Daniel Sutton, to inoculate in all parts of America south of Philadelphia.

Latham must have been a long way towards making his fortune when events conspired to put an end to the expansion of his business. Inoculators in New York and the more southerly counties had profited from the fact that the practice was still treated with suspicion further south, chiefly because of fears that the inoculated might start an epidemic. In January 1774, Latham became involved in anti-inoculation riots in Marblehead, a coastal town in Essex County, Massachusetts. Both Marblehead and the neighbouring town of Salem had approved the building of inoculation hospitals at a time when there was a great fear of smallpox breaking out in these close-knit communities. Although the authorities, the so-called Selectmen, had permitted the building of both hospitals, the population was fearful and suspicious.

Latham had been chosen as the inoculator for the Salem hospital, head-hunted from New York on the back of his reputation as a successful Suttonian. All went well initially, with the hospital taking in 137 patients in December 1773 and again in January, all of them inoculated by Latham. Whereas the Marblehead hospital had been funded privately, that in Salem was built by subscription, with a promise that once the fees of those being inoculated repaid the cost, subscribers would be reimbursed. But that was not to happen and Latham must have greatly regretted his move from New York.

At first the opposition was based on fear of contagion from those inoculated. Marblehead inoculation hospital, which had become known locally as Castle Pox, was burned to the ground. The ensuing attempts to arrest those responsible led to a stand-off between townspeople and the authorities, and the Salem Selectmen decided to close down their hospital. At this point Latham became a target of anti-British propaganda, specifically his association with the Suttons.[5] Patriotic New Englanders could not accept that a British inoculator was more accomplished than American inoculators.

One critic writing to the *Essex Gazette* referred to Sutton disparagingly as a 'blacksmith and farrier' who 'knew nothing of physic except for horses'.[6] Latham's record at the Salem hospital was questioned. It was said that his patients suffered more than those treated by rival American doctors who had their own, distinctive procedures. It was discovered that Latham's claim that his secret medicines did not contain mercury was false. Another letter in the *Essex Gazette* called him a 'Detested Imposter' because some of his patients had the symptoms associated with mercury. Other letter writers said Latham's patients had caught natural smallpox after they had been inoculated.

Joining the chorus of vitriol was the Salem hospital overseer Timothy Pickering, who had personally travelled to New York to offer the job of inoculator to Latham. He wrote a series of letters to the *Essex Gazette* signing himself 'A lover of truth', in which he accused Latham of a litany of crimes, the most serious of which was that: 'After wrestling from America the honor of its invaluable discovery' he was going to 'rob its worthy, learned physicians of their just profits'.[7] It was an American, so it was claimed, who discovered the use of mercury to alleviate the symptoms of smallpox, not Sutton, who anyway lied about using it.

The slanging match played out in the newspapers became so heated that readers pleaded for it to stop and for some real news to fill the column inches. In the brief time he practised at the Salem hospital Latham was said by his patients to have stormed about calling Pickering a 'damned rascal'. It is possible that in his rage he challenged his tormentor to a duel, writing to Pickering on 19 March 1774 to suggest he should meet him at a tavern or some other place that might be convenient. Pickering would not be drawn but signed off his tirade calling Suttonians 'a company of impudent imposters'. There was a suggestion that Latham should be hanged.

The attacks on Latham and Suttonian inoculation had little to do with methods of inoculation, but a great deal to do with the fact that Latham was an English interloper and, as the colonies formed patriot and loyalist camps, Latham was evidently in the latter. He did his best to appear neutral, but an English doctor practising an English form of inoculation was inevitably marked down as a loyalist wherever he went. In 1776, he set up a hospital in Great Barrington on Massachusetts Bay, advertising in his usual way in the *Connecticut Courant*:

> Sutton Inoculation
>
> Mr James Latham, Inoculator for the small pox acquaints the Public that their accommodations are now ready in the town, for the reception of strangers; attendance will be given by Mr Latham, or by one of his partners; that no person should be disappointed, upon the following terms, viz, For one person at a time, twelve dollars: for two persons or more at a time Ten Dollars . . . for which sum they are inoculated, dieted, lodged and attended. Great Barrington, Massachusetts Bay, 30 August 1776.[8]

This advertisement was soon followed by one in which Dr William Whiting, in search of patriot patients, informed readers that at his hospital they did not use the Suttonian method, but what he called the 'Dimsdation', after Thomas Dimsdale. On 4 July, a few weeks before Latham advertised in the *Connecticut Courant*, the colonies which had come together as the Continental Congress voted for independence.

Latham lived in a wealthy part of New York, in a community which was deeply divided. By conviction a loyalist, he struggled to make a living as an inoculator serving an increasingly hostile population. As his income fell, he turned his hand to business, for which he showed no aptitude. His plan to smuggle flour for the British Army led to a loss of £1,200 when his supplies were confiscated. This was a treasonable act and he relied on the support of friends to avoid arrest. He lost another £1,000 in 1783, shipping goods from New York to Philadelphia with permission from the British just as the long revolutionary war was nearing its end.

It is not easy to piece together the last years of Latham's life, which is recorded in fragments. He held on to his New York property at Livingston Manor, in which his wife Wilhelmina and sons James and Livingston had the benefit of a lease 'for and during their natural lives'. He returned to Quebec briefly but still practised in New York. Then, in 1790, there is a record of him becoming the surgeon at a British garrison in Kingston, Quebec. A year later he was granted 2,000 acres in Quebec by the British authorities, but there is no record of how this might have changed his fortunes. It seems he spent his last years alone as there is no record of his wife and children joining him in Quebec.

In a bathetic finale to his North American adventure as a Suttonian, he offered himself as an inoculator when there was an outbreak of smallpox in Quebec in the winter of 1796–7. He expected to inoculate local Mohawk Indians who had been hit by the epidemic. He waited with his lancet ready, but no Mohawk appeared.

10

An Imposter in the Family

Asserting his right to be regarded as the chief of the dynasty, 63-year-old Robert Sutton put an advertisement in the *London Evening Post* on 9 May 1771 to complain of 'many imposters who have assumed the Suttonian art of inoculation, and likewise my name'. He felt he was 'under the necessity of informing the public where my sons and partners reside to practise inoculation'. A lengthy list included accredited Suttonians not only in Britain, but in France, America and the Caribbean. Top of the list were all family: seven sons and two sons-in-law.[1]

A tenth family member might have been included: Daniel Sutton's father-in-law Simeon Worlock. He had been practising as a Suttonian since 1769, but he was not on the list. He was, in fact, the most blatant imposter ever to usurp the name of Sutton, safe in the knowledge that he could not be brought to book because he had quietly slipped across the Channel to Paris where, for several years, he enjoyed considerable celebrity.

Rachel, Worlock's daughter, was married to Daniel Sutton and living in the grand Sutton House when her father abruptly left London, never to return. Worlock probably picked up some of the secrets of the family business when staying with his daughter. If so, he did so surreptitiously, because the Sutton family were not pleased when they learned he was claiming to be a Suttonian inoculator in Paris. He certainly had no background in medicine. The wonder is that he won a reputation for his skill in both alleviating the symptoms of smallpox and as an inoculator.

Born in Antigua, Worlock was at one time a ship owner and merchant and was most likely involved in privateering – the polite term for piracy – in the Caribbean. It is frustrating that we know so little about Worlock's history until he appears in Paris around 1769, after which time his extraordinary exploits as a Suttonian imposter have been pieced together from French publications by Professor Michael Bennett.[2]

Worlock went to Paris in the hope of emulating the financial success of the Suttons, and presumably encouraged by the riches bestowed on Dimsdale in Russia and Ingen-Housz in Vienna. It is some measure of the Suttons' reputation that the very name could inspire confidence in a nation that remained resistant to inoculation. Worlock took what must have been a calculated risk in posing as a true exponent of the 'new method', for already established in Paris, claiming sole rights to Suttonian inoculation, was an English doctor, Joseph Power, author of a pamphlet *La nouvelle méthode d'inoculer*. Robert Sutton, Daniel's younger brother, also had a practice in Paris and was not at all pleased to learn that Worlock was masquerading as one of the family.

Worlock realised he could not simply announce his arrival in Paris with newspaper advertisements as he might have done in England. French doctors did not do that and it would have been too brazen anyway. Instead he appears to have had a cunning plan to slip quietly into Parisian society rather like a fugitive, taking any chance to demonstrate his imagined skills. According to Professor Bennett:

On arrival in Paris, he was able to use the Sutton names to set up a meeting with Antoine de Sartine, lieutenant-general of police. Assuming that Sartine would be curious as well as cautious, he spoke in terms of demonstrating the new method and cannily asked for someone to be assigned to oversee his practice. Sartine gave the task to Inspector Buhot, who was responsible for keeping tabs on foreigners in Paris. Sartine also nominated a member of the medical faculty, Dr Gardane, to follow Worlock at a discreet distance and learn all he could about the secrets of the Suttons.[3]

What Worlock lacked in medical expertise he made up for with sheer bravado. He relied on Inspector Bulhot to find him his first patients. These were selected from the small English-speaking community which frequented the Café Baptiste in rue de la Comédie Française: one was the daughter of Robert Godfrey, a glass painter, another a little girl who had contracted syphilis from a wet nurse and the third an Irish priest whose family had all died of smallpox and who feared he would be next. Somehow, Worlock managed to treat all three successfully and so impressed Inspector Bulhot that he asked Worlock to inoculate his own son.

At the Café Baptiste Worlock met an Irishman, Dr Sheehy, who was a qualified doctor who had been trained in Paris. In January 1770 they formed a partnership in which Sheehy would cover the expenses of a clinic in return for half of Worlock's earnings and a promise that he would be instructed in the Suttonian method. They were not allowed to practise within the Paris administrative boundary but found premises just outside one of the barrières which marked the limits of the city: it was close to where the cemetery of Père Lachaise is today.

Worlock promoted himself with anonymous letters to a number of publications reporting his achievements. The journal *l'Année Littéraire*, which had long campaigned for the adoption of inoculation in France, carried a number of glowing reports of his practice of what was termed the 'true Suttonian method', all of them clearly based on information provided by Worlock himself, or perhaps written by him.

He took any chance which came his way to impress. When his son, also Simeon, arrived in Paris, Worlock arranged for him to be taught French. When Simeon's tutor's son caught smallpox, Worlock was quick to apply his medicine and get the boy out into the fresh air. Here was further proof that he could treat smallpox as well as protect against it. This was written up in a report which said the boy had been snatched from *les bras de la mort*, literally 'the arms of death'.

Though he continued to report miraculous cures, Worlock was not making much money and his partnership with Dr Sheehy ended acrimoniously. He refused to pay Sheehy half his earnings, as agreed, arguing that a more conventional arrangement would have been payment of one third. According to Sheehy, Worlock refused to teach him the Suttonian method and, in fact, at this stage said Worlock claimed he was using his own method and was no longer Suttonian. When Sheehy tried to prosecute him for 3,000 livres, Worlock paid part of this sum and accused Sheehy of defamation. Frustrated, Sheehy contacted the Suttons who confirmed his suspicion that Worlock was a 'fraud and a charlatan'.

But that was by no means the end of Worlock. He left Paris in 1771 to practise inoculation in other parts of France, most extensively in Brittany. As he moved from one region of the country to another, he inoculated prominent families and retained his reputation as a skilled inoculator. But one or two doctors began to question his qualifications, guessing that he was really a quack. Salvation came with an opportunity to return to the Caribbean, with the recommendation of Antoine de Sartine the police officer who had first set him up in Paris and who was now a senior naval official. Slave traders were learning to inoculate their human cargoes in order to preserve their value. Worlock was well placed to take up inoculation in the wealthiest of France's slave colonies, Saint-Domingue, now Haiti. He sailed in 1774.

It seemed he was about to finally fulfil his dream of making a fortune. Before he left France for good, Worlock was involved in an argument with a French doctor who, in the pages of the *Journal Encylopédique*, had questioned his role in popularising inoculation in that country. There is no doubt that he had sufficient success in his treatment of smallpox and as an inoculator to justify this light-hearted riposte to his critics: 'I have opened a mine in your country, exploit it; live in peace, and don't quarrel with either the English or the healers.' On another occasion Worlock wrote: 'I am not a doctor nor a charlatan: I am a healer.' By that time he had renounced the association with his son-in-law which had enabled him to launch his career as an inoculator in 1769.

Sugar cane was grown and harvested in Saint-Domingue by an estimated 700,000 African slaves whose labour made the fortunes of a French colonial population of about 25,000. Worlock hoped to prosper here because plantation owners regarded inoculation as an investment, since it protected their slaves from outbreaks of smallpox, which were quite frequent and often devastating. Worlock was able to make a fortune with mass inoculations of the slave population. His son Simeon joined him and the two acquired property and 'aspired to landed gentility'. The elder Worlock reinvented himself as a scientist, sending observations to Paris and joining the elite, and possibly, Masonic academic society the Cercle des Philadelphes in Saint-Domingue in 1787. He became a Catholic and petitioned for French nationality. He died sometime before the slave revolt of 1791 in Saint-Domingue put an end to the country's colonial riches. It is not known exactly when he died, nor where he was buried.

His son Simeon fled to New Jersey to escape the bloody revenge on the island but died within a year. He is buried in an episcopal graveyard in Trenton with the inscription:

Beneath this marble lies the body of Mr Simeon Worlock, born and educated in England. He went at the age of 19 years to St Domingo where he resided until the insurrection in 1791, when he was forced to fly for safety with his family and friends, leaving behind an ample fortune. Having purchased the Bloomsbury estate near this place; departed this life on 23 July 1792 in the 35 year of his age . . . He lived beloved and died lamented.[4]

11

Inoculation for the Industrious Poor

In 1774, the same year that her father set sail to seek his fortune in Saint-Domingue cashing in on slave owners' enthusiasm for inoculating their slaves, his daughter returned to Antigua to convalesce. Family tradition had it that she did not take to the English climate. She had been away for several months when Daniel received the news that she had died on 25 February. She had left behind at Sutton House in Kensington two small children: a son, Daniel aged four and a daughter, Frances Dominicittie aged three. There is no record of who cared for them but there is some suggestion that family in Suffolk took them in. This family tragedy presaged a decline in Sutton's grip on the business he and his family had pioneered. Inoculation had come to be regarded as less of a luxury for those families who could afford it and more of an economic necessity to protect the 'industrious poor' in towns and villages.

It was not the end of the road for Daniel and the Sutton family, for their skills were still in demand. But the most lucrative business for which inoculators competed was now in the many schemes being promoted to offer inoculation to the poor. For those parishes that were prepared to pay for an experienced inoculator there was a great deal of choice. The rates the experienced inoculators charged varied considerably and there was a temptation just to go for the cheapest. But reputation still counted and a specialist drafted in was often preferred to the local doctors who were not always pleased to lose a lucrative commission. Both Daniel and his father had inoculated whole towns and villages before and would be an obvious first choice. Daniel was certainly considered when the village of Glynde in East Sussex was faced with an imminent outbreak of smallpox in 1767.

Glynde was in part of an estate inherited by the Rt Revd Richard Trevor in 1743. He had a reputation as a benevolent man – some thought him a little too generous as he allowed labourers and husbandmen free drinks from his brew house. George II favoured him, calling him 'the beauty of holiness', and made him Bishop of Durham. Trevor spent half the year at Castle Auckland, the bishop's northern seat, and half at Glynde Place. In his absence, the vicar of Glynde, the Revd Thomas Davies, acted as his agent while William Hodgson was his devoted steward, looking after all the interests of the estate and accompanying the bishop on his travels. His gardener was William Cordwell, whose wife brewed the bishop's beer.

It was the Revd Davies who first raised the alarm about smallpox. He wrote to Hodgson, who was then in London with the bishop, to warn that cases of the infection were being recorded only 10 miles away and there were many people from other parts of the county who had been inoculated, yet were allowed to wander about freely when they would have been infectious. The sheep farmer Richard Ellman was frightened to go to market but could not stay away as it would be the end of his livelihood. The same was true of Mr Tugwell the shoemaker.

The gardener's daughter was refused a post in service because she had not had the smallpox: it was a routine stipulation in advertisements for servants that they must have had the disease. On 28 February 1767 Davies wrote to Hodgson: 'I wish I could persuade our little Parish to do as Tunbridge Wells and Ryegate and such places have done i.e. to inoculate all in order to be clear of it in about a fortnight or three weeks.' Bishop Trevor gave his approval.

An inoculator who had made a name for himself in East Sussex was Dr William Watson who, in the year the Revd Davies approached him, had been appointed physician to the Foundling Hospital in London. Davies wrote to Hodgson that Watson had inoculated more than 2,000 people in East Sussex with 'equal success but less Physicking and more expedition than Sutton or his people'. Watson was not only quicker than Sutton, he was cheaper. 'The terms he offered to inoculate us I think is reasonable enough as he was very desirous of making an attack on Sutton.' Watson did not prepare his patients with any medications and used medicines only sparingly afterwards. His experiments with the orphans at the London Foundling Hospital confirmed him in his belief that most of the potions prescribed had little value. Watson's offer was to inoculate up to forty Glynde villagers for a total fee of 20 guineas and he would make a modest charge if there were more than that number.

Bishop Trevor gave permission for the stable house at Grand Place to be used as an 'airing' house for those who were inoculated and had to be kept isolated until their scabs had gone and they were judged to be no longer infective. There they followed the Suttonian practice of getting into the open air as much as possible. The villagers were divided into two groups so that work on the land could continue while one half were inoculated. It was a well thought out and well executed operation of which the Revd Davies was proud. However, the paupers confined to the Poor House were not included in the scheme and three of them caught smallpox. Of these, a woman pregnant with twins survived, but one of her newborn babies died.

Two hundred Glynde villagers were inoculated by Watson in the spring of 1767, most of them exhibiting only mild reactions and no fatalities. The Revd Davies was clearly pleased that his scheme had gone so well, and he was especially satisfied with Watson:

> There are at least a score of inoculating doctors advertising every week in the *Lewes Journal*, all in the newest Fashion, and I believe, as far as I can hear, all with the same success. For, if but anyone should happen to die, all the County would soon hear of it. Our doctor is above advertising and has not once appeared in print. I believe him to be as good as any of them, Sutton & Co not excepted.[1]

Though the Church had been opposed to inoculation when it was first practised in England, now that it had become popular it was not unusual for a rector or a vicar to be an enthusiastic supporter of it, as the Revd Davies was in Glynde. Some years later, in 1788, the *Gentleman's Magazine* published an account by the Hon. Revd William Stuart of a general inoculation he promoted in Luton, a small town with a much greater population than Glynde, but confined enough to make such a scheme feasible. Revd William was one of the eleven children of John Stuart the Earl of Bute and Mary Wortley Montagu, whose mother, Lady Wortley Montagu, had had her inoculated in 1721.

Grandson of a pioneer of inoculation (he possibly owed his very existence to his grandmother), the Revd Stuart carried on the family enthusiasm. He wrote:

> Towards the end of last summer a smallpox of the most malignant kind prevailed at Luton. Notwithstanding every care that human prudence could suggest, as to cleanliness, medicine and attendance scarcely more than half of our patients survived this dreadful disease; and though they were kept at some distance from the town, it was

found impossible to prevent the infection spreading. Alarmed at the danger I endeavoured to overcome the prejudice and fears of the people, and prevail on them to be inoculated.

Accordingly, in the course of three days a surgeon of the neighbourhood communicated the infection to 928 paupers, who were judged incapable of paying for themselves; and soon after to 287 more, mostly at their own charge. Of these 1215 only five died and those under the age of four months ... Meantime Mr Kirby and Mr Chase, the surgeons resident at Luton, inoculated about 700 of the better sort, with an equal success.[2]

The babies who died following inoculation were between 5 and 16 weeks old, their names and ages duly recorded by the churchwarden. This tragedy did not prevent the Revd Stuart judging the general inoculation a success, the more remarkable, he thought, because from his conversation with those who were inoculated, he learned that many of them did not take any of the medicines given to them. Nor could they be policed in a parish 39 miles in circumference so that some ignored the injunction to avoid strong liquor.

The Revd Stuart argued that the inoculation of hundreds of working people in Luton had paid for itself. In the nine years that he had been the vicar in Luton there were on average twenty-five deaths from smallpox each year. Caring for these patients cost the parish 2 guineas, exclusive of medical assistance. Nurses in the county were well aware of the dangers of attending smallpox sufferers and demanded double pay. Overall, the annual charge for treating smallpox victims would be 50 guineas. The same sum would pay for annual inoculations like that of 1788.

Even then, 50 guineas would not fully represent the cost of allowing the natural smallpox to take its course. 'If a labourer dies of smallpox his family must be supported. If a mother is lost the children must go into the workhouse.' In the workhouse they 'lose innocence, reputation, and that sense of independence which is the surest principle of industry . . . were inoculation generally practised it would lessen human misery, save many useful lives, and even promote that economy which many think the only object worthy of attention'.

The Revd Stuart had astutely recognised that the selling point for anyone wanting to promote a general inoculation was that it would benefit the economy not just by preventing a loss of trade that came with every smallpox epidemic, but also by preserving the workforce: the industrious poor, who did not have the means to protect themselves.

All those schemes for general inoculations which relied on the rich to pay for the cost of treating the poor emphasised that it was in their interests to do so. Invariably, it was the threat of an epidemic that persuaded a town to consider inoculation for everyone who would accept it. Faced with what was described in the *Hampshire Chronicle* as 'the present raging calamity', all the inhabitants of Winchester were summoned to the Guildhall two days before Christmas 1773. The mayor and aldermen proposed to debate 'the propriety of raising a fund by subscription for inoculating the inhabitants whose circumstances will not enable them to reap the benefit of that salutary art'.[3]

The proposal, said a report in the *Chronicle*, was greeted with 'unanimous approbation', being of 'such universal advantage to the trading part of this city and of such extensive benevolence to the poor'. And the poor were so grateful: 'Even the inferior orders of men, expressed, in a great degree, the pleasures which the most generous and liberal feel in imparting to the needy those blessings which the bounty of providence has impowered them to dispense.'

The appointed inoculator in this Winchester scheme was a Mr Smith Jnr, 'a gentleman who had practised for some time with Mr Sutton'. His charge was 5s 3d per head for poor people to be inoculated in their own homes. The committee responsible for the scheme obtained from the churchwardens and overseers an exact list of all the poor (parishioners and others) who had not had the smallpox and noted which of them agreed to be inoculated. The entitlement of those claiming free inoculation was checked, parish by parish, with the assistance of the ministers. All those who were given approval got a ticket which they took to Mr Smith, who would then submit it to the treasurers for payment. Servants whose employers could afford to pay for them to be inoculated, or who could afford it from their own pockets, were not eligible for a free ticket. However, if there was money left over they might apply.

The mayor and aldermen who promoted the scheme proclaimed in the *Hampshire Chronicle*: 'When this practice is thus rendered universal, it will be of the most beneficial nature that mankind was ever blessed with, and will always merit the greatest encouragement.' Up until that time the practice of only the 'rich' benefiting from inoculation was both unfair and dangerous. Once inoculated they could spread the disease to the poor and, practised in this limited way, 'the art is rather a curse than a blessing, and deserves every discouragement, nay every punishment, which it can possibly receive.'[4]

It was inevitable that Daniel Sutton, along with his father and brothers, would look for a way to cash in on this groundswell of enthusiasm for saving the industrious poor with schemes funded by charity and from local rates. However it was not at all in line with their regular business. They would carry out mass inoculations, as Daniel had done in Maldon, when asked, but their livelihood came from the charges they made for inoculating those who could afford the fees from their own pockets. Around 1770 there is a discernible shift in their approach which appears to have sent the Sutton family into some disarray. It began in February 1770, with Daniel Sutton advertising his new scheme for inoculating the inhabitants of London in their own homes. He was still then living in Sutton House, in fashionable Kensington, which was an incongruous address for launching a plan 'principally intended for the industrious poor; such as families of artificers, handicraftsmen, servants, labourers etc.'[5]

In October that same year the Suttons were advertising similar schemes in several parts of the country. They did not always give their Christian name, preferring to emphasise their kinship with Daniel. 'Mr Sutton, surgeon (Brother of Mr Daniel Sutton in London) at Mrs Wilkinson's in Rosemary Lane, Newcastle, proposes to inoculate the poor with the concurrence and support of the Nobility (and others) by subscription.' This was not so much a plea for compassion, as one directed at hard economic reality: 'At this time when the labour of the inferior mechanic and husbandman will scarcely provide clothing for their family . . . it is hoped that any proposal toward the benefit and preservation of that body of people will meet with due encouragement.'[6]

In effect, the Sutton brothers were hoping that the well-to-do would pay them to inoculate the industrious poor. So these were not schemes such as that in Winchester, which were promoted by aldermen and the gentry to allay the threat of an epidemic and who would appoint an inoculator of their choice. The Sutton model was purely commercial: pay us to inoculate those who cannot afford to pay themselves.

Daniel's proposal was ambitious, seeking to make inoculation in London 'universal'. It was a subscription scheme in which those contributing 1 guinea could nominate three patients 'and so on in proportion'. Daniel would sign the tickets himself and counter-sign them, which would 'entitle the patients for inoculation without further trouble'.

A patient who had a ticket would go to a reputable, Sutton-trained surgeon where they would receive medicines and instructions about how they should conduct themselves once they had been inoculated in their own homes. If there were any unusual symptoms they could call for

Mr Sutton or 'some of the Faculty concerned'. Subscribers could pick up their tickets from banks designated by Sutton in Pall Mall, Covent Garden, Fleet Street and Lombard Street in the City.

Despite the transparently commercial nature of his proposal, Daniel wanted to plead that his motive in proposing it was charitable: 'Mr Sutton has been urged to this undertaking by every motive of public spirit and humanity and has carefully digested and freed it from every reasonable objection. He flatters himself it will come recommended with such advantages to mankind as may induce the affluent and benevolent to support it, without whose alliance every act of public utility must prove ineffectual.'[7]

In Newcastle upon Tyne his brother proposed a subscription scheme where anyone paying 6 guineas or more could nominate twelve patients for inoculation, those paying 3 guineas could nominate six patients. 'Higher-class' people would pay between 3 and 10 guineas.

Daniel's scheme for offering inoculation to the mass of London's poor was clearly ludicrous. In October 1772, a Mr Sutton took out a notice in the *Public Advertiser* that he was moving from Kensington Gore to Goodge Street for the greater convenience of his patients. He was offering, in addition to his usual fees, free inoculation for the poor who were 'supported by charities'. He wanted to assure 'the labouring people' that inoculation would not take them away from their employment for long. He assured them that he had 'conducted many hundreds through smallpox with very little loss of time'.[8]

So Daniel had quit his splendid home in Kensington, or so it seemed. In fact, he was still there and in a rage. It was not his notice in the newspaper but that of his brother William, who had been living there with him for two years. There was a rapid response in the *Public Advertiser*: 'Daniel Sutton, respectfully informs the public that he continues to practise inoculation from Sutton House, Kensington Gore, as usual. He disclaims any connection with his younger brother William, of Goodge

Street, who publicly and privately has endeavoured to persuade the world that he is the Mr Sutton whose practice is to universally known and admired, when in fact it is Mr Daniel Sutton's.'[9]

Their father Robert intervened with his own notice, this time in the *Gazetteer and New Daily Advertiser*, describing himself as 'the sole inventor of the new method of inoculation' and advising the public that his son William was 'possessed of his art' and that there was no quarrel between his sons who were 'in a joint and perfect connection with each other'.[10] William soon moved on from Goodge Street to Rathbone Place around the corner, where he was joined by another brother (there is no record which) so that they could work together on his plan for 'inoculating the industrious poor and their families'. All they had to do was knock on his door in the morning to collect their medicines and arrange for their inoculation.[11] There would be no charges. In the same column of advertisements, Daniel said that anyone wanting to 'embrace the Suttonian method of Inoculation' could knock on *his* door at Sutton House before ten o'clock in the morning.

There is no record of what happened to Daniel's plan to offer sponsored inoculation to impoverished Londoners. What we do know is that his door at Sutton House closed for good sometime in 1766, when he moved nearer to the centre of town. He was still sufficiently well known for the *Public Advertiser* to report that, on 16 September, he had just returned to London from Cheltenham Spa and would start his winter 'campaign' near Leicester Square. He had moved to Leicester Street and took out an advertisement in which he 'desires no one may decline their application on account of his terms; those who cannot afford ten guineas for their inoculation . . . shall have the terms proportionate to their respective abilities'.[12] He explained his move into the heart of London as one of convenience for the industrious poor, who would have much less trouble getting to Leicester Square than to Kensington Gore.

In some of the advertisements that Sutton placed to encourage sponsorship for his 'universal' scheme, he made it clear that he was aware that there might be an objection that those who were inoculated would spread the disease. He stated that he was 'sufficiently aware that an objection may be urged against the utility of the scheme which is that, from the passing and re-passing of such number of inoculated persons through such a city the danger of a general infection might be dreaded.' These fears were unjustified, he argued, because at the infectious stage the 'disorder was reduced to such a benign state' and those inoculated would be at work in their own homes while infectious. This was wishful thinking: Daniel was now out of touch. The greatest difficulty of bringing inoculation to the industrious poor in large towns was that there was no way of isolating those with the infection from those who were unprotected. A randomly administered inoculation campaign was likely to do more harm than good.

This was understood by those promoting general inoculations, yet all they could do was plead that the poor who were inoculated did not mingle with crowds until they were free of the infection. Southampton, which in the eighteenth century was a popular resort for the well-to-do as well as a major port, conducted three general inoculations in the 1770s. Keeping smallpox at bay was exceptionally difficult because of the constant arrival of men from other parts of the world, while any outbreak was likely to frighten away the fashionable visitors to its resort. The town corporation put advertisements in the newspapers pleading for the inoculated to segregate themselves: 'All persons while under inoculation, or liable to convey the infection are expected to forbear going to any place of public worship, the markets, public houses, or any other meetings whereby the disorder may be communicated, the market people be deterred from bringing provision, or those who have not had the smallpox and may not choose to be inoculated, are alarmed; and the more effectually to answer these purposes, it is particularly requested that those who have not gardens will walk on the beach for the benefit of the air, and appear as little as possible in the streets and by no means on the turnpike road.'[13] Now that inoculation was widely practised, the greatest problem for those promoting it was this danger that it could spread the disease.

12

Saving the Nation

In the autumn of 1778 an English physician, John Haygarth, began a lively correspondence with doctors in both Britain and America who were interested in finding a way of overcoming the danger of inoculation spreading smallpox. Haygarth had circulated in the form of an *Inquiry* some ideas he had about the nature of smallpox infection and how it spread. Was there anywhere that might give a clue as to how the disease could be eliminated, he wondered. The answer came in a letter from a Dr Benjamin Waterhouse in Rhode Island, New England. Haygarth commented: 'At the time, I did not know, that smallpox had been excluded from any civilised country in the world: and was not a little rejoiced to learn . . . that what I conjectured to be practicable had actually been accomplished for a long series of years in Rhode Island.'[1]

Dr Waterhouse was born in Rhode Island just off the New England coast. It was an island then (later incorporated into the State of Rhode Island) 14 miles long and 7 miles wide. The main town, Newport, was busy with trade and shipping, but it was a tight-knit community which was able to monitor outbreaks of disease and take steps to control its spread. However, like some other counties in colonial America, it was opposed to inoculation. It kept smallpox at bay with a system of strict quarantine and isolation.

Those in the colony who wanted to be inoculated went south, principally to New York and Long Island. When they returned they had to discard the clothes they had worn while infectious. If anyone was suspected of suffering from smallpox they were visited by an inspector. If they were judged to have the disease they were taken away from their family by overseers to an island called Coaster's Harbour.

Dr Waterhouse, a professor of medicine at Harvard, recalled:

Formerly they carried the sick person in a box, in the form of a large chest, big enough to contain a small bed. The cover was perforated with holes sufficient to give the patient air. The box was put on an easy sledge and drawn by a horse, attended by the overseers to the shore, when the box and sledge together were put into a boat and in a few minutes the patient was in his hospital. When the inhabitants found that this formidable apparatus did more mischief, especially to timorous minds, than the disease itself, they dropt the use of the box and substituted a sedan chair.

If someone was found with an advanced case of smallpox, and it was thought not safe to move them, the whole street in which they lived was boarded up, warning advertisements put in the newspaper, and guards placed to prevent anyone coming near to the house. Dr Waterhouse made the point that these draconian regulations were regarded more as a popular custom than 'the restraints of the law'. The fact that the colony was free of epidemic smallpox when the disease raged elsewhere was reason enough for people to accept the regulations.

Rhode Island, which had a population of about 11,000, was, as Dr Waterhouse stated, 'the thoroughfare for all travellers from Connecticut, New York, the Jerseys, Pennsylvania and all the southern provinces'. A busy place, then, to protect from smallpox epidemics. The Rhode Island arrangements, though, would hardly be acceptable to the British people, though establishing something similar might have been Haygarth's dream. He was, however, a very cautious visionary, making his arguments carefully, not to say tediously, with case studies and the evidence of his many correspondents.

Haygarth was physician to the infirmary in Chester, a city in Cheshire which had suffered smallpox epidemics like every other town in the country. He was a firm believer in the value of 'the new method' of inoculation, but was troubled by the fact that it had not defeated the disease. He saw it as his first task to discover how the disease was transmitted from one person to another. There was still a widespread belief in the medical profession that in epidemics it was 'bad air', impregnated with the variolous poison, which was to blame. Some distinguished doctors believed that the infection could travel up to 30 miles through the atmosphere.

Haygarth sifted the evidence of his own experience and that of other doctors before he concluded that the infection could only travel through the air very short distances, not more than the space of someone standing close to another. It mostly likely travelled in droplets of water which were invisible but were contaminated with smallpox. In certain circumstances it could be carried in clothing that had been worn by those infected with smallpox. Proximity was the main danger which made poor families, crammed into a single room and often a single bed, so vulnerable.

It was important to know, for any programme of eradication of smallpox, when and for how long inoculated patients were infectious and therefore liable to spread the disease to those vulnerable to it. This was difficult to calculate because the time lapse between the moment of infection and the emergence of the pustules varied from one individual to another. So too, the final disappearance of the scabs left by the pustules. It was certainly a sufficient number of days for an inoculated person to spread the disease to other members of the family and anyone they were in contact with.

In the original approach of Robert Sutton and his sons, those who paid the fees for inoculation were routinely quarantined in the special houses hired to accommodate them. Those wealthy people inoculated in their own homes had room to isolate children and other family members. In a town like Chester, if a general inoculation called for in the face of an epidemic was to be effective, the poor somehow had to be persuaded to limit their contact with each other. Containment meant denying families who were infectious, either from natural smallpox or from inoculation, any contact with those who had not had the disease. For poor families this could mean not only a loss of wages but the expense of cleaning clothes that might be contaminated.

In 1774, Haygarth had been involved in the creation of a Smallpox Society in Chester, which aimed to carry out some such plan to make inoculation effective through isolation of the infected for a period of time. The society devised what Haygarth called the 'Rules of Prevention'. They were intended not only to minimise contact between the infected and the vulnerable, but also to make sure the infection was not lingering on anything, from clothes to a letter sealed by someone with smallpox. There was even a nervousness about any letter received which said something along the lines of : 'I am sorry to tell you I have been struck down with . . .'

The Rules of Prevention were policed by inspectors appointed by the society, who would visit homes in an effort to make sure that they were observed. It was not an easy task. Here, the rules are abbreviated:

1. No person who has not had smallpox should go into an infectious house.
2. No infected person, after the pocks appear, should go into the street or any frequented place.

3. Cleanliness was vital so no 'clothes, food, furniture, dog, cat, money, medicines or any other thing that is known or suspected of being daubed with matter 'should go out of the house unless it was washed and exposed to fresh air.'

4. The patient should not be allowed to approach anyone not protected till all their scabs have fallen off and all their clothes and possessions have been thoroughly washed, as well as the room they were in.

So that the inspectors would get an early warning of an outbreak of the disease, the Smallpox Society offered a reward for information provided by the public. Districts were identified where the infected families lived and promissory notes delivered offering rewards up to a maximum of ten shillings if they observed all the rules. In this way, the society hoped to contain an outbreak. Over three years it was found to be effective, reducing deaths from smallpox by half.

The society encountered considerable resistance, however: the endemic fatalism familiar to all those intent on saving the ill-housed poor of large towns of the virus. To their frustration, many of the poorest families rejected inoculation, preferring to allow their children to catch smallpox naturally. This was despite the entreaties of inspectors, who assured them the fatality rate from natural smallpox was at least twenty times that from inoculation.

On some occasions, the carefully planned defences of the Chester Smallpox Society were breached. The quartering of a regiment of soldiers in the town in 1780 led to an outbreak of smallpox which could not easily be contained. Despite the fact that a number of soldiers were clearly infected with smallpox, they wandered freely around the town. When one was challenged by an inspector he is said to have replied: 'Nobody takes care of me and I will take care of nobody.' The soldiers refused to have anything to do with Chester's Rules of Prevention. The Chester scheme was abandoned for lack of support from the townspeople. This was a great disappointment to Haygarth, but he did not abandon his ambition to find some way to stop the spread of smallpox.

Convinced that smallpox could only be transmitted over short distances, Haygarth reasoned that if those infected were moved to an isolation ward within Chester hospital, they would no longer spread the infection in the community and there would be little danger of them infecting patients in other parts of the hospital. An attic was converted into a 'fever ward', where patients were attended by nurses. The scheme worked but the nurses suffered.

Dispensaries for the poor, as an alternative to hospitals, were founded in London and other cities in the 1770s, offering some of the medical benefits of the well-to-do to the poor. These were akin to an early form of health centre where medicines would be dispensed and patients who could not go to a hospital were able to see a doctor. The Quaker philanthropist John Coakley Lettsom, who was involved in the formation of one such in London and in 1775, founded the Society for the Inoculation of the Poor in their own Homes. Anxious about the possibility of spreading the infection, the physician in charge, John Watkinson, collected evidence which he claimed showed that those inoculated with smallpox were so rarely infectious that there was no danger of patients returning to their own homes after the procedure.

This brought a broadside from Baron Dimsdale, which in the end was devastating to the whole project. The well-meaning promoters of the society would simply spread smallpox more quickly among the poor in their homes in the 'close alleys, courts and lanes'. According to Dimsdale, and his argument was not easily refuted, the only model that worked in London and larger towns was the specialist fever hospital or dispensary. They did nothing, however, to defeat smallpox, which the poor regarded with a fatalism that confounded the best efforts of those who urged them to protect their children.

John Haygarth continued to explore the possibility of bringing in the Rules of Prevention he had pioneered in Chester on a grand scale. After consulting physicians on both sides of the Atlantic, he produced in 1793 his ambitious *A Sketch of a Plan to Exterminate the Casual Small-Pox from Great Britain*. His 'sketch' ran into two volumes in which he meticulously laid out his reasoning over 570 pages. It was dedicated to King George III:

> History hath recorded many illustrious actions by your MAJESTY's ancestors, during a long succession of ages. Among them all, the most truly glorious, and in all its probable consequences, the most beneficial to mankind, was the introduction of inoculation into Europe in the year 1721.[2]

It was George I who, in 1721 offered to pardon the Newgate prisoners who volunteered to be inoculated: now, George III agreed to endorse Haygarth's grandiose plan for a national programme to eliminate smallpox for good through inoculation and isolation. The country would be divided into 500 districts, each administered by an inspector supported by 50 physicians, each one to cover 10 of the districts. Either George III himself or the Royal College of Physicians would be responsible for making the appointments. Overseeing the whole establishment would be supervising physicians based in London and three in Edinburgh. A new law would be enacted enabling those administering the programme to reward informants who reported outbreaks of smallpox or failure to follow the strict Rules of Prevention. Anyone who fell foul of these laws could be fined. Some histories, including a biography of Haygarth, claim that he revealed his authoritarian side when he suggested that any lawbreaker who could not pay the fine, or refused to do so, should be forced to wear in public a label reading: 'Behold a villain who has wilfully and wickedly spread the small-pox.' The source of this cannot be found in his original works and it is doubtful that the king would have endorsed such a proposal.

Any plan to make inoculation compulsory from the eighteenth century to the present day has failed. Inevitably, Haygarth was unable to persuade the medical profession of the feasibility of his plan, but he was anxious to emphasise what a huge benefit it could be to the British nation.

He asked his friend John Dawson, a country surgeon and self-taught mathematician, to look at the saving of life over the few years that the Chester Smallpox Society was active and to calculate what a similar reduction in the disease would be in Great Britain. Dawson was the son of a small landowner who made a meagre living as a shepherd on his father's farm until he was in his twenties when he demonstrated a remarkable mathematical ability. In 1756, when he was just 21 years old, he began to give lessons, becoming famous as the tutor of a number of the most successful students at Cambridge. Haygarth was one of his first pupils, when he was sixteen, and they remained friends until Dawson's death in 1820. Extrapolating from the Chester mortality figures, Dawson calculated that the annual survival rate would increase steadily so that after 60 years it would have saved nearly 200,000 lives in Great Britain.

In his ambition to rid the whole nation of smallpox, John Haygarth takes for granted that the safety and effectiveness of Suttonian inoculation had been demonstrated countless times. Its value was only limited by the political and administrative problems of making it universal. Haygarth makes no mention of Daniel Sutton or his family in his *Enquiry*, as if what they had achieved was too familiar to be remarked upon. Daniel Sutton did not fail to notice that his celebrity was on the wane.

13

Sutton's Swan Song

Once he had moved out of Sutton House, Daniel became itinerant, moving from one West End street to another in quick succession. In November 1775, it was reported that when travelling back to his new address in Leicester Street, near Leicester Square, around eleven o'clock on a Sunday at night, he was 'stopped and robbed of his money by two highwaymen, near Vauxhall Turnpike'. We can follow his meanderings in that vicinity with occasional references to the interest taken in him by thieves. In March 1776, his house in Lisle Street, Leicester Fields, was broken into by thieves who took house-linen, cotton counterpanes, toilet furniture, and a new black suit of velvet and 'other wearing apparel' to the value of £200. The report noted: 'The chest which contained them, with other household furniture, had been carried to the house but a few days before from his late dwelling house at Kensington Gore'.[1]

Daniel did not stay long in Lisle Street. In 1779, he announced that he had been 'engaged by the Governors of the General Inoculation Dispensary' and he had moved nearby to Southampton Street in Bloomsbury. Although he was still inoculating on his own account on his usual terms of 10 guineas, to have any kind of official post was out of character. Times had changed and he made it clear in yet another newspaper advertisement that he was well aware of the waning of his celebrity.

Announcing his appointment to the dispensary he felt it necessary to plead that he was the 'identical person who, in 1767 (by royal approbation) was complimented with a grant of the following honorary Patent for his singular and new method of inoculation'. This method, he claimed, was now 'very materially improved'. Once again the family coat of arms awarded to himself and his family was evoked.

Daniel had not been long in Bloomsbury when he was burgled again. 'Last night was stolen out of the house of Mr Daniel Sutton, Southampton Street, Bloomsbury, a quantity of men and women's wearing apparel. It is supposed the thieves got over the rails into the area and in at the wash house window whilst the servants were ironing in the kitchen adjoining.'[2] There is no record of Daniel re-marrying, but perhaps he had someone he lived with, as well as servants to do the ironing.

By this time, his father had moved to London and was setting up a practice nearby. An advertisement in January 1783 let the public know that 'the original improver of the Art of Inoculation and father of all the gentlemen of that name' had moved in with his son William in Charlotte Street. At the age of seventy-three he was still in business 'on the most reasonable terms'. There is no mention of his wife, Sarah, joining him in London, although she was certainly still living.

Five years after his move to London, Robert Sutton died at the age of eighty-one. The *Norfolk Chronicle* said 'he was the first of the name who practised inoculation with unrivalled success. He has left six sons who are very eminent in the above practice.'[3] He was buried in Thetford, Norfolk, not far from Framlingham Hall where he had practised as an inoculator. A brief obituary in the *Oxford Journal* stated: 'This was the gentleman to whom the world stands so much indebted for the very great improvements made in inoculation. He has left a wife who is also in her eighty-second year [that is, 81], six sons and three daughters with the whole nation to deplore his loss.'[4]

Daniel now took to advertising his services all over the country. His London addresses continued to change and there is no record of what his domestic circumstances were. In fact, the disappearance of newspaper advertising by the Sutton brothers not long after the father's death suggests that the name no longer had its former cachet. Now all inoculators were essentially Suttonian, whether they claimed any association with the family or not.

Why, at this stage in his career, Daniel chose to publish the account of his discoveries as an inoculator and to describe in some detail his once 'secret' technique is something of a mystery. He was 60 years old and he was surely aware that there was nothing much he could reveal that had not already been unearthed by rivals or rejected as unnecessary by detractors. Perhaps he wanted to make public the experiments he had made in his efforts to discover the mysteries of smallpox and how it attacked the human body.

He called his book, published in 1796, *The Inoculator; or, Suttonian System of Inoculation Fully Set Forth in a Plain and Familiar Manner.* There is no dedication, either to his father or anyone else. He makes the point on the frontispiece that he is the surgeon 'Who introduced the New Method of Inoculation into this Kingdom in the Year 1763'. In the preface he emphasises the importance of 'confidence in the operator' for those contemplating inoculation and presents his method of 'achieving excellency to young students in physic and surgery'.[5]

In a plaintive introductory 'advertisement' he complains that: 'I find it has been circulated that I am not the person who introduced the new system of inoculation . . . not the person who some years since resided at Kensington Gore . . . not person who had the honour of being presented with a special patent of arms . . . in short that for many years I had quitted my profession and was long since dead.'[6] Once again his citation for the coat of arms is rolled out like some obsolete certificate of excellence.

It is an odd lament because it was widely accepted that Daniel Sutton was the vital innovator, the Great Inoculator. If he was not better known now that his career was coming to an end, the only person he had to blame was himself, for he never joined any organisation and does not appear to have corresponded with other surgeons and physicians to compare notes. Unlike Dimsdale and Haygarth, he remained a loner supremely confident with his skill but uncertain of his status. Squabbling in the newspapers with other inoculators was not only unproductive, it sullied his reputation in the medical world.

The Inoculator did not break any new ground, but it did reveal some remarkable aspects of Sutton's quest to understand and therefore conquer smallpox. Among his observations on the most efficacious conditions in which to inoculate, he had discovered that the morning was better than the afternoon. This first came to his notice when he had inoculated 700 townspeople in a single day. 'About one half of them were inoculated before twelve o'clock and the other half were begun upon at half past three in the afternoon: They were all inoculated by my own hand, from the same individual subject without any selection of persons for either part of the day.'[7]

The treatment given in the morning was identical to that in the evening and there was no change in the weather. Yet those inoculated in the afternoon had, on average, five times the number of pustules than those inoculated in the morning. When he checked back through his notes on earlier inoculations he realised there was a pattern, and from that time on he favoured the morning for inoculation. This finding has been confirmed by recent research into the most beneficial times for modern flu vaccinations.[8]

Sutton had no clue as to why this might be: it is to do with a variation in the effectiveness of the immune system which he knew nothing about. He did his best to discover the secrets of smallpox but, after a series of bizarre experiments of a kind which would have had him locked up in the twenty-first century, he had to admit defeat:

> With respect to the peculiar miasma, or contagious essence, whatever it may be, should such a thing specifically and abstractedly exist (which as yet appears rather questionable) it is certainly of a nature too subtle, minute, and volatile, to be ascertained by any analysis yet known, nor have its contents been hitherto discovered by the help of our most perfect and compound microscopes.[9]

More powerful microscopes enabled the identification of 'germs', long after Sutton's death.

Haygarth had put a great deal of research into discovering how smallpox was passed from one person to another. Sutton, working entirely on his own, imagined he could crack the problem with a kind of makeshift laboratory. It is a shame there is no third-party witness to the first experiment he describes in *The Inoculator*. As a guinea pig, he chose a 'subject' who had not been inoculated or attacked by smallpox naturally, and who was therefore vulnerable to infection. For some reason, which he does not make clear, Sutton wanted to prove that you could not be infected with smallpox if you inhaled infected matter and filled your lungs with it. He wanted to bypass the 'lymphatics of the mouth'. It seems this was one of a series of tests to show that smallpox did not come from inside the body and then spread to the skin. He believed it was an infection 'of the skin'.

To this end he 'contrived a machine through which a person might inspire contagious air without danger of [it] being absorbed by the lymphatics of the mouth, in its passage to and down into the windpipe and the lungs'.[10] He does not give a more detailed description of this 'machine' but it must have been thrust down the throat of the hapless guinea pig. He (we assume it was a man) was instructed to breathe in highly infectious air from an inoculated patient. Sutton reasoned that if smallpox was absorbed through the lungs then his guinea pig would become infected. To his great satisfaction he discovered that, after several attempts, the man showed no signs of smallpox infection. Eventually, to prove the man had not already been immune, he inoculated him in the normal way and the disease took.

This was hardly conclusive, but he persisted. He wanted to see if he could infect someone with smallpox if the disease was incorporated into some pills which would be swallowed. The subject of this experiment, whoever they were, remained free of the infection. Sutton also tried both cool and tepid enemas (he used the archaic term clyster) 'strongly impregnated with both ripe and unripe pustules'. Again, the infection appeared to pass through the body without effect.

In his early days as an inoculator he tried the old-fashioned method of inserting the infection with deep incisions which, he said, often failed to propagate the disease. He wrote that he wanted to discover 'in what matter, and to what congenial parts of the body, the variolous particles did actually attach, so as to generate their increase'. His belief was that the smallpox poison only attached itself to what he called the 'true skin' and not to the flesh beneath. To test this he would make a deep incision in the patient's arm and place a piece of infected thread in it making sure it did not touch the skin. The infection did not take. He said he repeated this experiment several times with the result 'invariably the same'.

It was widely believed that smallpox emanated from the blood. Sutton doubted this and contrived what he regarded as a simple test. He took blood from a patient at the most infectious stage of the disease and, over a period of several days, used it to inoculate another patient. Repeated experiments showed no effect. It could not be blood then to which the 'variolous matter' became attached.

For his most ambitious investigation, Sutton turned pathologist. He wrote: 'It has been a generally received opinion credited even by some of the Faculty, and propagated as a truth that pustules do sometimes pervade the internal parts of the body; and this circumstance has been assigned as one of the reasons for such cases sometimes turning out fatally.' There was only one way to find out if this was true and Sutton awaited an opportunity to test the theory. 'A negro having on the ninth day died of the confluent small-pox, I had permission from his master to open the body: but on examining every part of the viscera and investiture [the peritoneum] not a pustule was to be seen, or any thing which had the resemblance of such an eruption.'[11]

These experiments were carried out over the years that he was inoculating, but he did not present them to the medical profession for comment and so they were never debated. When they were made public, reviewers of his book were not very impressed. The review in *The Critical Review and Annals of Literature* wondered why Sutton makes no mention of Haygarth and other published physicians and surgeons.[12] His experiments did not seem to make much sense or to further understanding of the disease. Sutton's opinion on the way in which smallpox invaded the body was opaque: 'some fecund influencing principle ... having a peculiar power over the variolous matter, does exist entirely upon and pervade the superficies of the true skin, between that and the scarf skin ...' At a stretch of the imagination you might say he had guessed at the existence of an immune system which had the effect of producing eruptions in its battle with the poison. But the discovery of that was such a long way in the future that it was of no value in 1796.

What Sutton had not anticipated, working as he did in glorious isolation, was that a new method of inoculation against smallpox was about to cause a sensation in the medical world both at home and abroad. It was, so its discoverer and his supporters claimed, much safer than that perfected by Sutton. There was no fundamental change in the procedure, just a change in the nature of the 'poison'. The crude matter taken from a smallpox sufferer for inoculation was replaced by an infection which appeared sometimes on the udders of dairy cattle and which, on occasion, was transmitted to the men and women who milked them. Known as cowpox, the pustules it gave rise to had a passing resemblance to smallpox. The infection was unpleasant but rarely fatal to people and yet used in inoculation it seemed to work just as well as smallpox itself.

The discoverer of this revolutionary method of inoculating was none other than Edward Jenner, the 8-year-old boy who had suffered from an archaic form of inoculation before the Suttonian revolution. After studying with John Hunter, a celebrated surgeon in London, Jenner had settled as a surgeon in Berkeley, the Gloucestershire village where he had grown up. He was a countryman, very observant and interested in wildlife. He had been elected to the Royal Society for his paper showing that young cuckoos, when they hatch, eject the eggs of the host bird. He debated on where swifts and swallows went in winter, a lively topic in his day. And, a follower of Sutton, he had experience inoculating against smallpox in the villages. The results of some general inoculations gave him the idea that an attack of cowpox might protect against smallpox.

The evidence was scant and his attempts to 'prove it' were few, but he took the decision to publish anyway, paying for the printing himself. Jenner had chosen to dignify what country people called cowpox by giving it a Latin name, *variolae vaccinae*, by which he meant 'smallpox of the cow'. There was no such thing, but the name stuck and his new method of inoculation was soon referred to as *vaccination*. For a few weeks he was despondent, as there seemed to be much scepticism about his claims. Then Jenner's discovery became an international sensation, with vaccine sought not just in Britain but in Europe and America as well. There were many in the medical profession who were sceptical of the claims made for it and regarded vaccination as what one detractor called 'Cowmania'.

14

Cowmania!

Vaccination was to conquer the world in a very short space of time, despite the fact that the research on which it was based was very limited and, in some vital respects, faulty. Jenner was ingenious and imaginative but he was not meticulous. This very soon became apparent as experiments were made with the vaccine. It did not always take effect and there were questions about the length of time it conferred protection against smallpox. However, Jenner's tract on cowpox could not be dismissed as the sensationalist work of an eighteenth-century quack. Its title was as sober as it was intriguing:

An inquiry into the causes and effects of the Variolae Vaccinae, a disease discovered in some of the western counties of England, particularly Gloucestershire, and known by the name of the cow pox, with observations on the small pox and on the subject of inoculation

There was one great problem when experiments with the effectiveness of cowpox vaccine were begun in earnest in many parts of the world: where to get the necessary infective matter. Smallpox was everywhere, so the supply for inoculators was assured, but vaccine was rare because cowpox was not a common disease and occurred only intermittently. It was known well enough among dairy farmers in Gloucestershire, where Jenner had his practice as a surgeon, but not in other parts of the country.

In the first printing of the *Inquiry*, Jenner expounded a theory that cowpox only occurred where men who tended horses also helped out at times with the milking. Horses were sometimes afflicted with an infection of their hooves called 'grease'. Farriers and grooms tending a diseased horse would carry the infection on their hands if they did not take care to wash them. When there was a demand for extra help with milking on the dairy farms, the men who tended the horses would help out and, according to Jenner, infect the cows. Equine grease then transmuted into bovine cowpox.

If that had been the case then Jenner's vaccine would have been rare indeed. As it turned out, his theory was nonsense. Jenner quietly dropped it after cowpox was found in London dairies, where there were no horses to infect them with grease. The wonder of Jenner's vaccine was that it worked. Not all the time, and not quite as effectively as Jenner imagined, but well enough to generate a huge demand for it. Vaccine soon became like gold dust: rare and apparently found only spasmodically in dairy-farming country, yet in demand in North America, where it was unknown, and throughout Europe, where it was not widely recognised.

At the Smallpox Hospital in St Pancras, London, Dr William Woodville had just published the first volume of his *History of the Inoculation of Smallpox in Great Britain* and a second volume was near completion when Jenner's research was published. Woodville abandoned his second volume and immediately went in search of cowpox. In the eighteenth century there were many dairies in London as there was no swift transport to bring milk from the countryside into town. Woodville found the disease in a dairy in Gray's Inn Road and immediately experimented with it among patients in the Smallpox Hospital. This was a near-disaster as the effect of his first vaccines seemed to resemble smallpox itself rather than cowpox. A smallpox hospital was the wrong place to test the effectiveness of vaccine inoculation.

George Pearson, a doctor attached to St George's Hospital at Hyde Park Corner, also searched out cases of cowpox in the capital's dairies and found supplies in St Marylebone and other places. Pearson also took it upon himself to conduct a survey of what was known about cowpox in the country as a whole, inviting reports on the success or otherwise of vaccine inoculation. He published his *Inquiry concerning the history of the cow pox* in 1798, in which he demonstrated that this disease was not unknown outside Jenner's Gloucestershire, and that it had long been suspected that those who had had it were protected against smallpox.[1]

Pearson received local reports sent in by clergymen as well as doctors; in fact, anyone who had an observation to make about cowpox. Pearson was convinced Jenner's discovery was genuine and, to encourage vaccination, he sent samples of cowpox vaccine to anyone who asked for it. Woodville and Jenner did the same, making no charge for the new drug. These were the days before modern forms of communication – no electric telegraph, no telephone, no ocean-going steamships, no internet – yet Jenner's vaccine went 'viral', being shipped around the world in a variety of improvised means of preservation.

A commemorative issue of the *British Medical Journal* of 1896, the centenary of Jenner's first inoculation using cowpox vaccine, retold the truly epic story of its rapid adoption around the world, encompassing Asia, Persia, most of Europe, Turkey, Spanish America, Russia and China. Jenner received from the United States an effusive letter of thanks penned by President Thomas Jefferson himself. From his Virginia estate, Monticello, on 14 May 1806, he wrote: 'You have erased from the calendar of human afflictions one of its greatest. Yours is the comfortable reflection that mankind can never forget that you have lived. Future nations will know by history only that the loathsome small-pox has existed and by you has been extirpated.'[2]

Jenner had sent a copy of his *Inquiry* to one of the indigenous North American peoples and was honoured with a speech given in 1807 at a Council of the Five Nations at Fort George in what was then Upper Canada. 'We shall not fail to teach our children to speak the name of Jenner; and to thank the Great Spirit for bestowing upon him so much wisdom and so much benevolence. We send with this a belt and a string of Wampum, in token of our acceptance of your precious gift; and we beseech the Great Spirit to take care of you in this world and in the land of spirits.'[3] The chiefs of the Five Nations, which included the Mohawks, signed the address with their tribal symbols.

The search for cowpox lymph remained a problem, and finding and maintaining supplies involved an international effort. There was in the eighteenth century a medical grapevine which connected the more forward-looking doctors and scientists in Europe and North America, many of whom, whatever their nationality, had studied in Edinburgh or Leiden and worked for a time in the more famous London hospitals. The *British Medical Journal* remarked, a little smugly: 'It is interesting to observe how great an influence the English nation has had in diffusing the benefits attaching to a discovery which was wholly of English origin.'[4]

A young Swiss doctor, Jean de Carro, after studying medicine in Edinburgh, decided to practise in Vienna, where he soon had a thriving private practice and moved in the most fashionable circles. He was alert to all new ideas in medicine and, intrigued by Jenner's *Inquiry*, was keen to get his hands on some vaccine. A friend from Geneva, Alexander Marcet, who had also studied in Edinburgh was then, in 1799, a lecturer in chemistry at Guy's Hospital in London found him a supply. Marcet knew Jenner, who gave him some infected thread which was sent to

Carro in glass vials. With this, Carro conducted the very first vaccination in what was then the Austro-Hungarian Empire.

Later, Carro got most of his vaccine from Italy, where Luigi Sacco, after a long search, had discovered cowpox in the northern region of Lombardy. Sacco, who practised as a doctor in Milan, visited Lugano County Fair on the border with Switzerland in the autumn of 1800. Two of a herd of cattle showed signs of cowpox in the early stage of the disease, as described by Jenner. He followed the herd to Cremona, waiting for the pustules to develop, and collected lymph when they ripened. From these two cattle, Sacco managed to distribute thousands of vaccines to many countries.

Carro became an enthusiastic promoter of vaccination and was involved in introducing it to Germany, Poland, Hungary and Russia. In the summer of 1800, a British diplomat in Vienna invited him to a banquet, an occasion which led Carro to introduce vaccination to Turkey, whose practice of inoculation for smallpox had inspired its first practice in Britain. At the banquet, Carro met the parents of Lady Elgin, wife of Lord Elgin, then ambassador to the Ottoman government in Constantinople (now Istanbul). When the Elgins learned of Carro's enthusiasm for vaccination they asked for some vaccine to be sent to them. On a second attempt they succeeded in vaccinating their infant son. Lady Elgin became a vaccinator herself in Turkey, treating the ex-pat community. Had she lived, Lady Mary Wortley Montagu would no doubt have been gratified to learn that England returned to Turkey a new, and supposedly improved, version of the technique that she had promoted in 1721.

The Elgins later took vaccine to Salonika in Greece in 1802, from which a thousand children were vaccinated: soon after that, vaccination was established in Athens. It was the beginning of the international vaccination odyssey much appreciated by Edward Jenner, who was moved to send Carro a small gift, a snuff box inscribed: 'Edward Jenner to Jean de Carro, as a token of his esteem and gratitude for Dr Carro's first having diffused the practice of vaccination on the Continent and for transplanting the vaccine matter into Asia.'[5]

Almost simultaneously, vaccine was being introduced to France, Malta and Gibraltar in the Mediterranean, and Spain. The Russian Empress Maria Feodorovna called for vaccine to be sent to her, but there would be no need for an inoculator like Baron Dimsdale to make the journey to Moscow. Vaccine, preserved on ivory lancets and threads, was sent from Breslau in Prussia, arriving on 1 October 1801. The girl from the Moscow foundling home who was the first to be inoculated with it was named Vaccinoff and given a pension for life. She was sent on to St Petersburg in a royal coach where vaccine was taken from her to inoculate all but the youngest children in the foundling home.

This was the start of a widespread vaccination campaign in Russia. In the absence of any local source of vaccine, the only way to propagate it was 'arm to arm', and many children like Vaccinoff were used as carriers. In 1802, the empress sent Jenner a thank you letter (written in French), with a diamond ring enclosed. In return, he sent copies of his original *Inquiry* and later publications.

Nowhere was the clamour for vaccine in the first few years of 'Cowmania' more extraordinary than in France, which had been at war with Britain since 1793. In 1796, Napoleon Bonaparte won a series of stunning victories before he seized power in 1799, but the desire to benefit from Jenner's vaccine over-rode all military considerations and desperate attempts were made to acquire supplies.

A professor at the University of Geneva had travelled to London to get hold of a copy of Jenner's pamphlet and a partial translation appeared in *Bibliothèque britannique*, a magazine published in Geneva to make English literature available to a French audience. Other magazines printed extracts and a young Swiss doctor, Antoine Aubert, translated

Woodville's account of his pioneering experience with vaccination at the London Smallpox Hospital. The Society of Medicine in Paris was cautious but decided to run a trial with three foundlings.

Aubert got the vaccine from Woodville, but when it failed he was despatched to London to see how it was done. There he was welcomed by Woodville who allowed him to vaccinate in the Smallpox Hospital. Two more attempts in Paris failed, at which point Woodville decided to return to Paris with Aubert. They first sailed to Hamburg and from there took a neutral ship to Boulogne, where they were delayed for a day. Woodville took the time to vaccinate some children there. By the time he reached Paris, his vaccine was ineffective. Vaccine from the children treated in Boulogne provided fresh lymph and finally Paris achieved its first success.

The French had already established a Central Committee of Vaccination, a foundation which served as a repository for vaccines, a model for countries around the world adopting vaccination. It was a great commendation for Jenner when the committee confirmed, in 1803, that his discovery was genuine. A Napoleonic medal commemorating vaccination (but not Jenner himself) was struck in 1804. Such was Jenner's reputation with the enemy that he was able to appeal success-fully on several occasions for the release of prisoners held by the French. He also wrote letters of commendation for travellers abroad which had the status of a passport. John Baron, Jenner's friend and biographer quotes one such:

I hereby certify that Mr A the young gentleman who is bearer of this and who is about to sail from the port of Bristol on board the *Adventure*, Captain Vesey, for the island of Madeira has no other object in view than the recovery of his health. Signed Edward Jenner, Member of the N.I. of France Berkeley, Gloucestershire, July 1 1810.[6]

It is often said that Napoleon had his armies compulsorily vaccinated. While he was in favour of vaccination it was Napoleon's ministers who were responsible for the introduction of vaccination to France. It was never compulsory in the army.[7] However, in 1811, when his son was born, Napoleon had him vaccinated before he was baptised and the news that the emperor endorsed the new inoculation greatly increased its popularity.

Getting vaccine to Spain's vast American territories presented perhaps the greatest challenge of all in the global adoption of Jenner's discovery.[8] Vaccination had begun in Spain in 1802 and was encouraged by the royal court. A demand for it inevitably arose in the colonies, which were plagued with epidemics of smallpox. There was a doubt that vaccine, preserved in some way, would retain its potency on a voyage across the South Atlantic.

The solution was to take on board a group of boys – orphans of course – who had not had smallpox and to vaccinate them 'arm-to-arm' in sequence during the crossing. A ship was fitted out for the expedition, with doctors and nurses on board to look after the children, who were all boys from a foundling home. They were vaccinated two at a time with the lymph of the first of them 'harvested' about ten days later from their arms and used to vaccinate the next two. En route, the ship stopped at Tenerife in the Canary Islands and began vaccination there. After calling at Puerto Rico and Caracas, the expedition divided, a ship heading down to South America, while the ship that had left Spain sailed to Florida and Yucatan.

This odyssey, which was named the *Real Expedición Marítima de la Vacuna* (the Royal Maritime Vaccine Expedition), could not have been contemplated without 'arm-to-arm' propagation of the vaccine. But in the long run it had many disadvantages. There was the exploitation of the children, the risk of infection with other diseases in the continuous transfer and perhaps a limited supply of orphans. After much experimentation, the solution to the creation of vaccine was provided by the cow. Attempts to infect cattle with smallpox were not very successful, but infecting one calf with cowpox taken from another did work. The calf had its hide scarified, that is, scratched, and the pox infection rubbed in. In this way one calf could supply up to a thousand doses of vaccine. In Paris, the infected animal would be walked around the streets so that vaccinations could be performed on the spot.

Within a year of the publication of Jenner's *Inquiry*, the advertisements of Suttonian inoculators were being superseded by those of the vaccinators. One of the earliest vaccinators to set up in business was Henry Jenner:

INOCULATION of the VACCINE DISEASE

   or COW-POX

Mr Jenner, surgeon, nephew of Dr Jenner, discoverer of the Inoculation of the Cow-Pox, having, in conjunction with Dr S experienced the most extensive opportunities of practising the inoculation of the genuine disease, and of observing its effects, proposes to extend its advantages to the inhabitants of Bath and its vicinity.

It is incontrovertibly demonstrated by some thousand instances, of the validity of which Mr J. is ready to adduce the most satisfactory evidence that the *genuine* Cow-Pox, effectually prevents the reception of the Small-Pox; that it is never fatal, produces little or no indisposition, and is unattended with eruption. It is also never followed by the Scrofulous, and other diseases which often succeed the Small Pox.

Mr Jenner may be referred to at No. 10 Miller's Court, Bath.[9]

What was the '*genuine* cowpox'? There were infections to which cows were susceptible that appeared to be cowpox but were not, and these faux afflictions did not produce a vaccine which provided a defence against smallpox. The many early failures of vaccination were attributed to this misdiagnosis of the cow's infection. Jenner produced an illustration to identify true cowpox on an infected udder. Then there was the much greater problem of vaccine contaminated with smallpox, which occurred at the Smallpox Hospital in London with fatal results.

However, 'Cowmania' was a wild, worldwide clamour for a medical innovation which had not been subject to more than cursory, and not always satisfactory, scrutiny. Suttonian inoculation, on the other hand, had stood the test of time and there were those who doubted if vaccination offered a great improvement. One, not surprisingly, was Daniel Sutton himself. He must have watched the craze for vaccine with mounting astonishment. Yet he did not join in the fierce debate between the Suttonian inoculators and the vaccinators. He simply indulged in his favoured means of getting his point across, an advertisement in the newspapers:

Cow Pox no security against Small Pox

Mr Daniel Sutton, No. 43 Red Lion Street, Red Lion Square, author of 'The Inoculator: or, the Suttonian system of Inoculation', assures the public that, by a process, peculiar to himself perhaps, he is enabled in most instances after a certain period from vaccination, to communicate the small pox to such subjects as have been deemed effectually vaccinated by the most celebrated Vaccinators.

No fee will be charged in case of failure.[10]

Typically, Daniel does not say what this 'process peculiar to himself' is. It might have been useful to other inoculators, but it probably would have made little difference to the international will for cowpox inoculation to work. As it was, nobody was seeking Sutton's expertise anymore.

In his *History of Immunology* Arthur Silverstein asks:

Why was it that the practice of inoculation made such slow progress despite its Royal Patronage, whereas vaccination gained substantially worldwide acceptance and use within a very few years, though lacking any official backing at the outset? There was ... no substantial difference in the quality of the initial data on safety or efficacy ... The difference may well rest less on the force of scientific evidence than on a variety of unrelated social factors, as is often true of medical vogues even today.[11]

15

Jenner's Debt to Sutton

When newspapers first learned that there was a new way of protecting communities from a smallpox epidemic, they saw it as an improved version of the kind of inoculation with which they were familiar:

INOCULATION

New Discovery

Inoculation, which has been found so highly beneficial in preserving the human species from the ravages of Small Pox, has been recently very much improved. The custom of communicating the disease by taking it from the patients who laboured under it, is now beginning to be abandoned by a number of surgeons in the Metropolis. The *cow pox* has been found to supply the infection in a most favourable way to those who are inoculated.[1]

Once regarded as shocking and dangerous, the use of the surgeon's lancet to provide protection against smallpox had become routine by the end of the eighteenth century.

In *The History of Immunology* Arthur Silverstein noted:

In 1722 such measures as smallpox inoculation were restricted to a relatively small class of the educated and landed gentry ... But throughout the eighteenth century the concept of public health spread fairly widely, as was witnessed by the health and welfare of the underprivileged. Indeed inoculation itself helped pave the way for vaccination, since much of the population saw the latter technique as an improved version of one already in use. Thus, by the start of the nineteenth century, we may tentatively suggest that society as a whole was better prepared than it had been seventy-five years earlier to accept what appeared to be a significant medical advance against the dread of smallpox.[2]

But would Jenner have discovered the protective power of cowpox even if there had been no inoculation before vaccination? That is unimaginable. Nobody, however observant and ingenious they were, could have contemplated injecting a cattle disease into the arm of a child unless it was an alternative to the familiar and routine procedure of inoculation with smallpox matter. In his account of how he made his discovery, Jenner attributes it directly to his experiences as an inoculator. And yet, there is a persistent myth, or fairy tale, which has this country surgeon inspired not by the hard evidence gleaned from mass inoculations, but the uncommonly pleasing complexion of milkmaids in Gloucestershire.

In one version of this imagined moment of inspiration, Jenner notices that dairy maids in Gloucestershire never have their good looks damaged by pock marks, which suggests they are immune to smallpox. Perhaps this is because they are liable to be infected with a disease called cowpox locally. In another, related, version, the people of Gloucestershire, a county full of dairy cattle and renowned for its cheese, have an age-old belief that a bout of cowpox will protect against smallpox. Jenner takes note and decides to put this belief to the test.

John Baron, in his biography of his friend Jenner, tells a story that might just be the origin of the pretty milkmaid legend. Baron recalls that

Jenner told him that when he was a young surgeon he had overheard a milkmaid saying she could not catch smallpox because she had had cowpox. The thought was lodged in Jenner's memory. The biography appeared after Jenner's death, so there was no chance for him to confirm or deny the story. Perhaps it was Baron's way of suggesting that Jenner's ideas about cowpox went back a long way, as he was in his fifties before he put the idea to the test.

Jenner himself would almost certainly have protested that he arrived at his belief in the protective power of cowpox by a much more considered and systematic method. Jenner made clear he believed it was the fact that inoculation had become commonplace and was carried out extensively in towns or villages, that gave rise to his suspicion about the protective power of cowpox.

There is no mention at all of pretty milkmaids in his account of his discovery. Men were infected with cowpox too, if they helped out with the milking. Nor did Jenner believe there was an age-old tradition among country people about the protective attributes of cowpox.

In a pamphlet on the origin of vaccine inoculation published in 1801, Jenner wrote of cowpox:

> a vague opinion prevailed that it was a preventive of the Small Pox. This opinion, I found, was comparatively new among them; for all the older farmers declared they had no such idea in their early days – a circumstance that seemed easily to be accounted for, from my knowing that the common people were very rarely inoculated for the Small Pox, till that practice was rendered general by the improved method introduced by the Suttons.[3]

Before widespread inoculation, no farm worker or dairy maid would *know* if they were protected from smallpox. And not all dairy maids were infected with cowpox, which broke out intermittently, so there is no reason to believe their good looks (if that was the case) were a result of immunity to smallpox.

Jenner, like all experienced inoculators, discovered that one or two of the people he treated did not develop the symptoms of smallpox, which indicated they must have been immune. John Haygarth in Cheshire believed that one in twenty of those seeking inoculation would discover they were immune and saw no relationship with any other disease. In fact, if Haygarth's estimate was right, there must have been reasons for immunity other than a previous infection with cowpox, as it was not widespread enough to have an effect in every region.

Daniel Sutton encountered patients who appeared to be already protected for no apparent reason, and it troubled him. He wrote in *The Inoculator*:

> It sometimes happens that persons, unconscious of having had the small-pox, present themselves for inoculation; and they, no less than the operator, under such unforeseen and embarrassing circumstances, must be mutually disappointed in their expectations. Hence a second, third, or even a fourth operation has, from time to time, been insisted upon by one or the other, but with no better effect; and each, in his dissatisfied state, takes leave of the other.[4]

Sutton thought it most likely that those who were already protected had had smallpox at some time in their lives without realising it. He had devised a simple way of discovering if a patient was immune without putting them through the tedious business of special diets and medicines. He would insert his lancet in the usual way, just under the skin, slant-wise, no deeper than a sixteenth part of an inch and examine the skin just above the lancet when raised up. If it looked pale he would judge that person immune. 'Should the patient be informed on the instant of being inoculated that he has already experienced the disease it will give him the clue and the motive for enquiring among relatives or others as to the fact thus unexpectedly declared.'[5]

It did not occur to Sutton that those who resisted inoculation with smallpox might have suffered a similar disease. This is not surprising, as any connection was much more likely to be recognised by a country doctor like Jenner, who was familiar with the lives of many of his patients. Sutton was more like a lone ranger, taking his skills wherever he thought they would be most sought after and where he could earn the most money. When he lived at Sutton House, Kensington, or any of his other London addresses, he would know very little about the lives of the patients who knocked on his door. If he was familiar with any families they would likely have been well-to-do and be ignorant of cattle diseases.

Jenner was well aware that his position in Berkeley in Gloucestershire was an especially favourable one for a study of the possible links between cowpox and smallpox. Whereas Sutton would have no way of knowing if a patient who resisted the inoculation had at some time in the past had smallpox, Jenner felt he could be certain of it. 'Had these experiments been conducted in a large city, or in a populous neighbourhood, some doubts might have been entertained; but here, where population is thin, and where such an event as a person's having had the smallpox is always faithfully recorded, no inaccuracy in this particular can arise.'[6]

By his 'experiments', Jenner meant a series of case studies collected over a number of years. When general inoculations in villages and small towns were undertaken, it was invariably the case that some patients could not be infected with smallpox. They would have no idea why they were resistant when the rest of the family inoculated at the same time were not. They would be asked if they had ever had smallpox. Jenner believed that if they had suffered from it this would not have escaped notice in a close community. Even if they had had the infection as an infant and could not recall it themselves, someone in the family or village would know. He reasoned that there must therefore be another explanation for their resistance to smallpox. By no means were all those Jenner judged immune milkmaids.

The first example he gives in the *Inquiry* is the case of Joseph Merret, a gardener working for the local squire the Earl of Berkeley. He and his family presented themselves at a general inoculation in 1795 to stave off a threatened epidemic. After several attempts, it was impossible to infect Merret. Though he lived with his family, one of whom had the smallpox 'very full', he was not affected by exposure to the disease. Jenner does not say exactly when or how it was discovered that Merret had had cowpox twenty-five years earlier, in 1770, while working as a farmhand.

It would have been a distant memory, but cowpox was an unpleasant enough disease when caught 'naturally' from the diseased cow to stick in the memory. Jenner gave a description of it:

The system becomes affected – the pulse is quickened; and shiverings, succeeded by heat with general lassitude and then pains about the loins and limbs, with vomiting, come on. These symptoms, varying in their degrees of violence, generally continue from one day to three or four, leaving ulcerated sores about the hands, which, from the sensibility of the parts, are very troublesome . . . the lips, nostrils, eyelids and other parts of the body are sometimes affected with sores.[7]

The implication was that, although Merret knew very well he had had cowpox, he did not think it would have made him immune to smallpox. Whenever he encountered someone who resisted the inoculation infection, Jenner would ask, first, if they had had smallpox before and, second, if they had ever had cowpox. Almost invariably, anyone showing resistance to the inoculation would recall an attack of cowpox.

Jenner presented several case studies where the cowpox infection dated back a number of years, as he was concerned to show that the protection afforded was not short-lived. There was the tradesman, John Phillips, who had had cowpox when he was 9 years old and who was inoculated with only a mild effect at the age of 62. A woman called Mary Barge had been regularly employed as a nurse with smallpox patients without becoming infected. An attempt to inoculate her resulted in a rash which died away after a few days without smallpox pustules developing. She had caught cowpox thirty-one years earlier, while working for a farmer.

One surprising discovery Jenner made was that it was 'well known' that farm hands and dairy maids who had survived a smallpox infection appeared to be protected against cowpox. This knowledge was important, as an outbreak of cowpox could seriously disrupt the working of the farm because those affected would be off work for several days. Those who had had smallpox could be drafted in, sure that they would not get cowpox at all, or only in a very mild way.

These, and all the other histories Jenner presented to support his case for vaccine inoculation, could not have been performed without Suttonian inoculation. And when Jenner came to attempt his first practical experiment with the vaccine, he was already an experienced Suttonian inoculator. He believed the key to Sutton's success was the manner of inserting the infective matter with the lancet barely breaking the skin or drawing blood. That is how he chose to perform his first vaccination.

Cowpox came and went in Gloucestershire, and Jenner had to wait for it to appear before he could carry out his experiment. His time came in May 1796, when he treated a local woman, Sarah Nelmes, who had become infected with pox from an infected cow called Blossom, which she had milked when she had a scratch on her hand from a thorn. Jenner noted: 'A large pustulous sore and the usual symptoms accompanying the disease were produced in consequence.'

On 14 May 1796, he 'selected a healthy boy, about eight years old, for the purpose of inoculation of the cow pox'. He does not give the name of the boy in his *Inquiry*, nor does he say how he 'selected' him for the experiment. Like Sarah, the donor, the boy was from a local family, a desperately poor one in his case. Jenner would have known him and felt confident that he had never had smallpox.

His name was James Phipps and he was to become, unwittingly, the most celebrated guinea pig in the history of medical research. It is not clear whether or not Phipps and his family were aware that the incisions Jenner made in his arm were to insert cowpox rather than smallpox, nor whether they were offered any financial incentive: poor children were fair game in medical research at the time. In his *Inquiry*, Jenner described the reaction Phipps had to cowpox: 'On the seventh day he complained of uneasiness in the axilla [arm pit], and on the ninth he became a little chilly, lost his appetite, and had a slight headache. During the whole of this day he was perceptibly indisposed, and spent the night with some degree of restlessness, but on the day following he was perfectly well.'[8]

That was the first part of the *vaccine* experiment. It is not clear, but it is likely, the final 'proof' of the effectiveness of vaccine was carried out by his nephew Henry. On 1 July, Phipps was inoculated with smallpox in the Suttonian manner with the result Jenner had hoped for: the boy's reaction was typical of that of someone who was resistant to smallpox. A few months later Phipps was inoculated again, with the same gratifying result. Encouraged by this first attempt at vaccination, Jenner experimented with the transfer of the cowpox infection from one child to another.

Daniel Sutton would not have heard of Jenner before the *Inquiry* was published to such a storm of publicity. But then few people outside the dairy country of Gloucestershire knew anything of Jenner either. If he was known at all, it was for his research into the cuckoo. As the Royal Society had accepted Jenner's paper on the cuckoo, he anticipated that they would publish his account of his researches into cowpox as a protection against smallpox in their *Philosophical Transactions*. But his paper was rejected. No official reason was given, but it is almost certain it was turned down, not because it was regarded as far-fetched but because there was insufficient evidence to support Jenner's conclusion. Jenner had the confidence to ignore this rebuttal and to publish himself.

The belief that vaccination was just a better form of inoculation was encouraged by the claim that it required no preparation, no diets or medication, more akin to a modern vaccine. And Jenner was happy for anyone to learn his method, which, in essence, was no different from Sutton's unintrusive use of the lancet. Baron, in his biography of Jenner, wrote that, in addition to the large number vaccinated by professional gentleman in different parts of the world, 'it is but proper to commemorate the services of many ladies and gentlemen in England who particularly distinguished themselves by their efforts in the cause'.[9]

Philanthropic zeal had taken inoculation to the poor through hospitals, dispensaries and general inoculations of whole towns and villages. The nobility were invited to sponsor these. But there was nothing to compare with the great upswelling of support for vaccination. Women, many of them aristocratic, not only promoted the new inoculation, they practised it themselves. There had never been any regulation of inoculation and there was none when Jenner performed his first vaccination. He was not opposed to unqualified vaccinators: in fact he encouraged them, instructing them in the technique of selecting the lymph and employing the lancet.

Baron wrote:

> notwithstanding the clamour which was raised against unprofessional vaccinators ... they rendered good service to the cause ... I have often heard Dr Jenner speak with satisfaction of the conduct of the ladies. Miss Bayley in particular managed the process with much skill and perseverance. In order to detect any cases of failure that might occur in her practice she would give a reward of five shillings to any one who could produce an instance of smallpox after vaccination performed by her. Out of 2000 cases, only one was brought to claim the reward.[10]

Vicars, who mostly opposed inoculation in the early days, now embraced vaccination with enthusiasm. Foremost among them was the Revd Rowland Hill (no relation to the Penny Post man), a flamboyant preacher. According to the Revd Hill's biographer, when he learned about Jenner and vaccine, he befriended him and announced: 'this is the very thing for me!' Daniel Sutton had paid the Revd Robert Houlton £200 a year to preach in his little church in Ingatestone, whereas Jenner had the proselytising services of Hill for free. Wherever he preached he would announce at the end of the sermon: 'I am ready to vaccinate to-morrow morning as many children as you choose; and if you wish them to escape that horrid disease the small-pox, you will bring them.' It is estimated that the Revd Hill personally vaccinated 10,000, 'coaxing the little frightened children in the most good natured manner.'[11]

In their last years, Sutton and Jenner, the two most influential practitioners in the century-long history of inoculation, would sometimes live close enough to each other in London to have knocked on each other's door. Sutton's home in Hart Street (now Theobalds Road) was a stone's throw from Bedford Street and Great Russell Street in Bloomsbury, where Jenner stayed when he was in town. There is no record of them ever meeting, nor is there any record of a correspondence between them. If Sutton ever wrote any letters they are not preserved. Jenner, on the other hand, was an inveterate letter writer and yet there do not appear to be any addressed to Sutton.

Jenner had made passing reference to Sutton in his *Inquiry*, but as soon as the clamour for vaccine made him an international celebrity he condemned Suttonian inoculation as archaic and dangerous. In 1809, he wrote from his home in Berkeley to his friend Dr Thomas Charles Morgan in London: 'Opposition to vaccination seems dead – at least in this part of the world we hear nothing of it. Thro' a vast district around me, I don't know a man who ever *unsheaths that most venomous of all weapons, the variolous lancet*.'[12] This was the very 'variolous lancet' that he had unsheathed himself over many years; the same wicked lancet that had inoculated the thousands whose experience informed his research into cowpox, and the very same he had used to test the effectiveness of his vaccine on young James Phipps.

Extraordinary that Jenner could dismiss with such contempt what, for nearly half a century, had been considered a hugely beneficial medical revolution: inoculation against smallpox. The very notion that Suttonian inoculation was 'venomous' and the lancet used was a 'weapon' was wicked, intended no doubt to enhance the claims for vaccine. And the belief that there was little or no opposition to vaccination was wishful thinking. Jenner might have heeded Sutton's warning that his vaccine was not failsafe. But then it was some years before it was thoroughly tested.

In 1802, in the full flush of 'Cowmania', Jenner, with help from his influential friends, petitioned Parliament to provide him with a stipend of £20,000 in recognition of his introduction and promotion of vaccination. At this point his gainsayers searched the country for examples of vaccination which pre-dated Jenner's experiments, and they found them.

In 1774, there was an outbreak of smallpox in a part of Dorset. A prosperous farmer, Benjamin Jesty, chose not to have his wife and children inoculated in the Suttonian manner, but instead to seek out a cow with cowpox. According to Jesty, he had two servants who had had cowpox, from which he had also suffered, and found that they were all three safe to nurse people suffering from smallpox. He reasoned, therefore, that he would infect his family with cowpox. He marched them across the fields on a round trip of several miles to take cowpox directly from an infected cow. He made an incision with one of his wife's stocking needles and inserted the cowpox. It is not clear if he thought it was safer than conventional inoculation or he simply wanted to save the cost of an inoculator's fees.

The children fared well enough but his wife became seriously ill and he was forced to call a doctor, which is how the story became known locally. It did not re-emerge until a committee in Parliament was debating whether or not Jenner should be given the stipend for his discovery of vaccination. Jesty was invited to London by George Pearson, who had turned from Jenner's champion to his chief antagonist, a quarrel over precedence which soured their relationship. The Jesty story was judged interesting but irrelevant: it had no bearing on the later discovery of vaccine.

Nevertheless, MPs were not entirely convinced that vaccination was an improved method of protecting against smallpox. They voted for him to have half of the money by a small majority. In 1807, Parliament was petitioned again and, following a favourable report by the Royal College of Physicians, the second £10,000 was granted. Putting the case for Jenner, the Chancellor of the Exchequer Spencer Perceval made it clear that vaccination was regarded not as something entirely new but an improvement on Suttonian inoculation. He reasoned:

> If they assumed, that the inoculation for the small-pox was a benefit to mankind, they might then be able to estimate how much greater a benefit this discovery was, which, as appeared by the report, was a certain security against the small-pox. It appeared, that of those who had that disease naturally, one in six died, whilst of those inoculated for that disease, only one in 300 died. But of 164,381 cases of persons vaccinated, only three had died, which made the mortality only one in 54,741.[13]

This second tranche of the stipend was voted through with a majority of just thirteen. But that was not quite the death knell for inoculation.

16

The Battle for Vaccination

The worldwide excitement for Jenner's vaccine in the first flush of Cowmania promised a new era in which parents would clamour to have their children protected by this new and safe form of inoculation. This would have realised the dream of John Haygarth, who had imagined a national scheme and dismissed it on the grounds that it was unenforceable. But vaccination was not greeted with the enthusiasm that might have been anticipated. In the first decade of the nineteenth century, vaccination was favoured over inoculation by Parliament and by a majority of the medical profession, but not by the public. Faced with the threat of an outbreak of smallpox, the offer of free vaccination was often turned down in favour of tried and trusted inoculation in what was now the 'old method'. Authorities realised that, to be effective, a general inoculation had to offer the public a choice of Sutton or Jenner.

A letter published in the *North Devon Journal* of 8 May 1828, signed anonymously as 'A friend of the medical profession', described just such a dilemma:

In a town in the North of Devon a vagrant's child was taken ill of the Small Pox in the natural way, and as soon as the eruptions maturated, medical gentlemen began to inoculate, without any previous consultation. The magistrate, very properly, as soon as he heard of it, called a meeting of the inhabitants, and it was by them determined to have all the poor children vaccinated and inoculated at the public expense; option was given to the paupers to have either . . . there were about three hundred and eighty paupers inoculated and vaccinated, and about two hundred and fifty others; the proportion inoculated was about eight to one; in the neighbouring parishes some thousands have been inoculated and vaccinated, and I believe the proportion inoculated is at least twenty to one vaccinated.

The writer complained:

I conceive that a more methodical method of bringing vaccination into disrepute could not have been adopted – many families lived in the same tenement and court, where some were vaccinated and others inoculated at the same time. If vaccination failed, or the lymph proved to be of a spurious kind, they were liable to take infection from those inoculated, and to have the smallpox in the natural way, which, by the uninformed, would have been solely attributed to the fallibility of vaccination.[1]

The great danger of inoculation with smallpox matter was that it could very easily start an epidemic if someone at the infectious stage came into contact with those who were unprotected. This was widely recognised and not seriously disputed. On the other hand, it had become clear long before Jenner's death in 1823, that vaccination often failed. Evidence also emerged that that it did not confer life-long immunity. From the point of the individual, Suttonian inoculation was the more reliable and, in most cases, no less troublesome than vaccination. On the other hand, from the point of view of public protection, vaccination, even with its frequent failures, was superior: the drawback of its unreliability was far outweighed by the knowledge that it could not cause an epidemic.

In 1793, the forward thinking Dr John Haygarth had imagined a nationwide programme which would ensure that all children were inoculated with no possibility of the disease spreading. But he realised it would be impossible to implement. The structure was not there and the public would not tolerate the draconian measures which would be necessary to make it work. Exactly the same dilemma confronted those who now, in the early nineteenth century, realised that vaccination would never get rid of smallpox unless the great majority of children were given the protection as infants. Newspapers carried the annual reports of the National Vaccine Establishment, founded in London by Jenner and others to promote the cause. In May 1821, presenting their findings to the Home Secretary Robert Peel, they wrote:

My Lord, it is with great regret we announce to your Lordship, that the small-pox has occasioned the loss of many lives in various parts of the united kingdom, since our last report ... great prejudices still persist against vaccination and ... the benevolent designs of the government are still far from being accomplished.

This Board has laboured incessantly to set forth the comparative case and safety of the indisposition of vaccination and the difficulty and danger of smallpox whether occurring naturally or occasioned by inoculation.[2]

The Royal College of Surgeons had sworn that its members would not agree to inoculate with smallpox even if they were asked to do so. It reported:

This good example has been followed by most of the respectable practitioners in the country; though some of them, we are sorry to say, have lent themselves improvidently to this injurious practice. And we find that the multitude in many places have been so infatuated as to accept the professed services even of itinerant inoculators, in spite of their gross ignorance of all disease, and of the rudeness and ineptitude of the instruments which they employ to insert the poison.[3]

While doctors in Britain found it hard to convince the public that they should adopt vaccination for their own good, in Europe there was much less resistance and deaths from smallpox were falling. As the *Quarterly Review* of 1826 put it, quoting a Scottish doctor frustrated by his efforts to stamp out quackery in medicine: 'England is a free country, and the freedom which every free-born Englishman chiefly values, is the freedom of doing what is foolish and wrong, and going to the devil in his own way.' This, said the *Quarterly Review*, 'strikingly exemplified the present state of vaccination in Great Britain, compared with its state in other countries in Europe'. Those who were not vaccinated were prevented by governments from being confirmed, attending school, taking up an apprenticeship or getting married. The doctor continued: 'Small pox inoculation was prohibited; if it appeared in any house that house was put under quarantine; and in one territory no person with small pox was allowed to enter it.' In England it was a free for all.[4]

A doctor had come up with an ingenious solution which he had put in a letter to the president of the Royal College of Physicians. Dr Ferguson suggested that children should first be vaccinated, as this would temper any reaction to smallpox, and then inoculated to ensure long-term or lifetime protection from the disease. They would not spread the infection and yet they would be safe. In this way, the intransigence of the

British public could be overcome. But there is no evidence that this was ever put into practice.

By the 1820s it was evident that Britain was being left behind in the control of smallpox. The *Quarterly Review* spelled it out:

> In Copenhagen mortality had been reduced from 5500 during 12 years to 158 in 16 years. In Prussia it had been reduced from 40,000 annually to less than 3000 and in Berlin only 5 persons died of this disease ... In England, on the other hand – in England, the native country of this splendid and invaluable discovery, where every man acts on these subjects as he likes, crowds of the poor go unvaccinated; they are permitted not only to imbibe the smallpox themselves, but to go abroad and scatter the venom on those who meet them.[5]

One of the many accounts of the disastrous consequences of the refusal of the 'lower orders' to accept vaccination was published by John Cross, a surgeon in Norwich. In 1819 he witnessed in this Norfolk town one of the worst epidemics of the early years of vaccination. Cross described Norwich in the early nineteenth century as a generally wholesome place, which experienced intermittent outbreaks of smallpox. From 1813 there were five years where the disease disappeared altogether. Very few of the population had taken the opportunity to get their children vaccinated or inoculated when, in June 1818, smallpox reappeared. It had been brought into the town, it was believed, by a girl who had travelled down from York with her parents. There were only a few cases of smallpox in the town before the end of the year and two deaths.

A chemist had inoculated a few people, but the disease did not spread until the following February. Then, a charity school was infected and smallpox appeared all over the town in what Cross described as 'the most extensive destruction of human life that has ever ... taken place in Norwich in the same space of time from any other cause than the plague'. Deaths from smallpox began to rise alarmingly to 73 in May and peaked in June with 156 deaths, falling gradually to 142 in July, 84 in August and 42 in September. In total, from January to December 1819 there were 530 recorded smallpox deaths. The greatest number of victims, 260 in all, were infants under the age of 2. There were 132 deaths of 2- to 4-year-olds and 85 of 4- to 6-year-olds. In fact, all but five of those who died were children. Cross, who himself attended 200 of those afflicted, estimated that around 3,000 out of a population of about 40,000 had been infected and this was 'confined almost exclusively to the very lowest orders of people'.[6]

This was despite the fact that Norwich had introduced a novel scheme a few years earlier in an attempt to lure or bribe the poor to accept vaccination. A Dr Rigby had persuaded the local authority, the Board of Guardians, to offer 'half a crown' to every poor person who brought a certificate to them from a surgeon confirming that they had 'satisfactorily gone through the cow-pox'. In ten weeks, more than 1,300 claimed their reward. But when the threat of smallpox receded, more and more of the poor spurned the donation. Only the danger of another epidemic would drive them back to vaccination. Only eleven rewards were claimed in 1815. There was a sharp rise in 1816 to 348 and then a falling away again. In the epidemic year of 1819, vaccination rewards claimed peaked at 359 in August and had fallen to zero by December.

Cross could not tell how many had been inoculated during the epidemic months. Out of 93 surgeons who replied to his request for information about their practice, 38 had performed some inoculations where patients refused vaccination or families expressly asked for it. Cross concluded: 'Medical Men, however, inoculated comparatively few cases during the year of the epidemic. The greatest inoculators were the parents of poor children, farriers, blacksmiths, tailors, shoemakers and old women.' The practice of inoculation was now regarded not just as dangerous, because it might aid the spread of smallpox, but because it produced a high mortality among those who chose it: hearsay evidence collected by Cross suggested that more than fifty deaths could be attributed to this discredited practice.

It is evident that the vaccinators, taking their cue from Jenner, wanted to cast Suttonian inoculation, which had once been at the very pinnacle of medical advance, in as grim a light as possible. It is likely that artisans and 'old women' inoculators in 1819 were not too fastidious in their methods and perhaps the Suttonian art had been forgotten. But then in its early days, vaccination had been embraced enthusiastically by amateurs with Jenner's encouragement.

In 1840, the medical campaign against inoculation with smallpox finally succeeded in persuading Parliament to ban it. A bill proposing the creation of a framework for providing free vaccination across the country was carried with an amendment proposed by Thomas Wakley, MP for Finsbury and the founding editor of *The Lancet*. Inoculation was banned, with the penalty of a prison sentence for those who refused to comply with the law. Had he lived long enough, Daniel Sutton could have been prosecuted for practising the art he had perfected.

The national scheme of free vaccination was administered by the Poor Law Guardians, managers of the hated workhouse and grudging distributors of financial relief to the poor. It was pointed out by Wakley, among others, that this did not bode well for the success of the Vaccination Act: those it was intended for were opposed to vaccination and would hardly welcome a doctor appointed by the Poor Law Guardians. It was obvious within a few years that it was not going to work. So, in 1853, the decision was taken to make it compulsory for parents to have their children vaccinated by the age of three months.

The protests began soon afterwards. An anti-vaccination pressure group was formed and soon martyrs to the cause were accepting jail sentences rather than comply with the law. And now that Suttonian inoculation was out of the way, all attention was focused on vaccination. And it was clear that Jenner's wonder 'drug' was not what he and his supporters claimed. Whereas inoculation had provided life-long protection against further attacks of smallpox, vaccination's protection was relatively short lived. Before this was recognised in Britain, other countries in Europe had begun the first programmes of re-vaccination. There was a long-standing problem, too, with the supply of vaccine. 'Arm to arm' propagation was now regarded as unhygienic and inconvenient, and it risked spreading syphilis.

Frustration with the opposition to vaccination, led to laws being tightened up in a series of Acts of Parliament giving magistrates the power and responsibility to prosecute parents who did not comply with the law. At first there were fines and then prosecutions, with those sent to jail for a month treated as martyrs for the cause by the anti-vaccination movement. In February 1877, hundreds gathered in the Oxfordshire town of Banbury to greet two local men who had served one-month jail sentences for defying the law on compulsory inoculation.

A torchlight procession around the town was organised with an effigy of Jenner in tow. The idea was to set fire to him that night, but this was delayed as one of the men who had been in Northampton jail was released later than expected. When he returned to Banbury, a second procession was hijacked by some young boys who took delight in throwing missiles at Jenner's torched effigy. A disgruntled farmer wrote to the *Banbury Guardian* to complain that the ammunition the boys used was dug up from his vegetable garden.[7]

There was widespread coverage of the Banbury protest, which encouraged defiance of the Vaccination Acts. This reached a peak in 1885 with a massive demonstration in Leicester, which was again given widespread coverage. The *Aberdeen Press and Journal* of 28 March 1885 reported:

Between 2000 and 3000 persons assembled at Leicester on Monday to protest against the prosecution of 5000 defaulters under the Compulsory Vaccination Acts. Delegates were presented from all parts of the country and banners were carried in the procession from all parts of England and the Continent.

The procession, which was over two miles in length, started from the market place amid great enthusiasm, and the streets were lined with thousands of spectators. The procession was of an extraordinary character, and included a gallows, upon which an effigy of Jenner was hung, while a cow and a horse were exhibited as specimen sources of vaccination, and a coffin drawn upon an open bier as the result of the operation. Afterward the Acts were burned in the market place in presence of a vast concourse of spectators. Fifty thousand persons were present and great enthusiasm prevailed.[8]

The *Graphic* commented on the mass opposition in Leicester:

Jenner, the discoverer of the cow pock, whom we were taught to regard as one of undoubted benefactors of the human race, has just been hanged in effigy by the intelligent inhabitants of that flourishing borough. His offence, of course, was what used to be regarded as his chief merit, namely that he was the inventor of that abominable and detestable practice, vaccination.[9]

The National Anti-compulsory Vaccination League, which had been founded in 1874, proved to be a successful pressure group, publicising cases of children supposedly harmed by vaccination and of parents fined or sent to jail for refusing to comply with the law. In response, the government established a Royal Commission on Vaccination which spent six years collecting evidence on the effects of inoculation and vaccination. The commission considered the success or otherwise of smallpox inoculation which it judged to have been 'very general' in the latter half of the eighteenth century. 'It was especially so during the last quarter of the century, the increase being at least largely due to the "improved methods" of inoculation introduced by one Sutton in 1763, and known as the "Suttonian method".'[10]

Sutton's achievement, the commission noted, was to infect patients with smallpox so mild that it hardly caused any discomfort, was rarely if ever fatal, and yet conferred immunity from future attacks. The conclusion was that Suttonian inoculation had benefited the rich and the well-to-do more than the poor and that it had 'a double influence, one favourable and the other unfavourable as regards small-pox; and, owing to the conflict between these two influences, it produced but little effect upon the prevalence of or mortality from smallpox.' However, the commission concluded that the balance of probability was that it did not increase the prevalence of smallpox as some vaccinators had claimed.

The commission acknowledged the many drawbacks of vaccination: the frequent failure to confer immunity, the spreading of diseases to children and the widespread resistance to compulsion. But the evidence was that the incidence of smallpox had declined and that, on balance, it was successful. Bowing to the demands of the National Anti-compulsory Vaccination League, it was recommended that parents should be allowed to declare themselves 'conscientious objectors' and avoid prosecution. This became law with the 1898 Vaccination Act and around 250,000 parents applied for exemption orders.

Even in the years just before the 1914–18 war, it was estimated that only about half of all infants were vaccinated against smallpox. Yet, the disease appears to have lost much of its virulence and there were few deaths. It was only in 1948, with the founding of the National Health Service, that the legal obligation on parents to get their children vaccinated was lifted. Vaccination against smallpox ceased altogether in 1971. It was a fantastic triumph for medicine, which was followed shortly after by the elimination of smallpox 'in the wild' entirely, the one and only human virus ever to be eradicated.

17

·⊙══════⊙·

Sutton and Jenner
The Legacy

Just a few newspapers and magazines devoted a paragraph recording Daniel Sutton's death at the age of eighty-three at his home in Hart Street, Bloomsbury, on 3 February 1819. The *Gentleman's Magazine* acknowledged the debt the world owed to him:

> Mr Sutton, as appears by his 'System of Inoculation' published in 1796, first attempted in 1763, the innovation on the system of inoculation for the smallpox, which he afterwards put in practice to an immense extent, and with extraordinary success at Ingatestone, and subsequently in the Metropolis, and various parts of the Kingdom. The benefits which the world has derived from Mr Sutton's practice have been duly appreciated, and will cause his name and memory ever to be recollected with respect and honorable distinction.[1]

It was not to be. Abraham, in his biography of John Coakley Lettsom, wrote: 'Daniel Sutton died forgotten, having lived for over twenty years after Jenner's great discovery made his contribution to the advancement of science, and the preservation of life, no longer necessary. Had Jenner's discovery never been made, Sutton's statues would be everywhere.'

There was no institution to carry Sutton's name into the era of vaccination, his family was scattered and none had any connection with medicine. There is not a single Sutton memorial in London or anywhere in the country, or, as far as is known, in the rest of the world. His importance in the defeat of smallpox would not be acknowledged even now if it were not for the interest historians have taken in eighteenth-century medicine in recent years.

In 1987, John Smith, an Essex archivist, published *The Speckled Monster*, a historical account of smallpox in that county, in which he unearthed a good deal about Daniel Sutton's influence. He subsequently wrote accounts of the lives of Daniel and his father Robert which are now, belatedly, in the *Oxford Dictionary of National Biography*.

The late David Van Zwanenberg, formerly a surgeon attached to Ipswich hospital in Suffolk, published an article in *Medical History* on 'The Suttons and the business of inoculation' in 1978. He credited Daniel with devising the minimally invasive method of inoculation which was subsequently adopted by vaccinators throughout the world eradication campaign.

Dr Peter Razzell, a social historian with a special interest in eighteenth-century demography, discovered the Suttons while researching the cause of the steady rise in England's population from the 1770s. In his book, *The Conquest of Smallpox*, first published in 1977, he challenged the received wisdom that medicine was so primitive in the eighteenth century it could not have had any effect on mortality. Sanitary improvements and a rise in births following an increase in the rate of marriage were assumed to have been the most important influences on population growth. Dr Razzell unearthed such a wealth of evidence on inoculation and its widespread practice that he was able to contend that it must have played a part in population increase. The key figure was Daniel Sutton, who made inoculation popular.

There was certainly contemporary support for the view that Suttonian inoculation had had a hugely beneficial effect on health in the eighteenth century. The *Gentleman's Magazine* in 1796 was emphatic:

The increase of people within the last 25 years is visible to every observer ... Inoculation is the mystic spell that has produced this wonder. Some time between 1738 and 1743 (I speak from memory) the smallpox was so severe at St Edmundbury the assizes were twice, if not three times, held at Ipswich. During that term, it was said, that the town had been deserted, deprived of the fifth part of its inhabitants: there were no markets, and the town was avoided as the seat of death and terror. This was no more than a common calamity at the time ... It is now 30 years since the Suttons, and others under their instructions, had practised their skill in inoculation upon half the kingdom and had reduced the risk of death the chance of one in 2000. Hence the great increase in people.

The incidental advantage has been that the present race is much handsomer than formerly: the beautiful lineaments of Nature, and her celestial texture of the skin, are inviolated. That this has been in favour of chastity I dare not aver.

The article was signed with the pseudonym 'Candide'.[2]

If this author were correct in his argument, and the rise in population was crucial to the 'take off' of the Industrial Revolution in the eighteenth century, then Daniel Sutton's historical significance would be greatly enhanced. However, as the Final Report of the 1896 Royal Commission concluded, the record of smallpox mortality is too patchy and slender for any conclusions to be drawn about the role of inoculation in either increasing or reducing population. That debate continues.[3]

While vaccination was hailed as much safer and more successful than Suttonian inoculation, smallpox continued to attack communities throughout the nineteenth century and Edward Jenner's reputation waxed and waned. His death in 1823 was mourned throughout the world, and many British newspapers carried lengthy obituaries. The *Gentleman's*

Magazine began a five-column tribute: 'With unfeigned sorrow we have to announce the death of Edward Jenner, the discoverer of Vaccination'.[4] His nephew Henry, one of the first to inoculate with cowpox, found him lying on the floor in his library, unconscious. Henry bled him and applied blisters to his feet while his friend Dr Baron, later Jenner's biographer, was sent for. But Jenner could not be revived and died in the early hours of the morning on 16 January 1823. He was 73 years old.

Just after Jenner died, there was a request to the government to grant him a state funeral with burial in Westminster Abbey. But nothing came of it. Later, Robert Peel, then Chancellor of the Exchequer, explained in the House of Commons that the government was sympathetic to the idea of a state funeral for Jenner but the family had said they preferred a private ceremony. Dr Baron claimed that Peel omitted to say that the family were told they would have to pay for a state funeral, the cost of which would have been prohibitive for all but a very wealthy family. So Jenner was buried in St Mary the Virgin churchyard, Berkeley, where his father had once been the vicar, in the village where he had lived for most of his life. His admirers from Cheltenham attended and it is said that James Phipps was among the mourners. Jenner had given him and his family the lease of a small cottage for life.

No London doctors attended. Some of his friends and admirers appealed for money to pay for a memorial of some kind, but there was little enthusiasm. After months of appeals a young English sculptor, William Sievier, still in his twenties, agreed to take the commission for whatever money was raised. His statue was placed in Gloucester Cathedral in 1825. It has Jenner posing in academic robes clutching an honorary degree, or diploma, he was awarded in 1813 by Oxford University. Baron recalled Jenner feeling uneasy wearing the doctoral robes at the presentation in Oxford, as he was quite unfamiliar with the rituals of academia. He had at least one memorial soon after his death where Sutton had none.

It was as well for Jenner that he did not live to witness the anti-vaccination campaigns of the later nineteenth century in which his effigy was burned. And it was long after his death that those seeking to commemorate his achievement managed to have a fitting memorial created. A subscription was raised in 1858 to pay for a statue of Jenner, but there was little enthusiasm. The project, promoted by the sculptor William Calder Marshall, would have failed if it had not been for the generosity of Jenner's admirers abroad. The United States was the most generous contributor, followed by Russia, with Britain a grudging third. Queen Victoria gave permission for Jenner to be placed on a pedestal in Trafalgar Square and Prince Albert, a vaccination enthusiast, performed the unveiling. The dedication read simply 'JENNER'.

The siting of the statue was not universally approved. Thomas Duncombe, an MP, complained: 'Cow pox was a very good thing in its proper place but it had no place among the naval and military heroes of the country.' The satirical magazine *Punch* ridiculed him and imagined, in a bit of verse, what Jenner's response might be:

England, ingratitude still blots
The scutcheon of the brave and free
I saved you many million spots
And now you grudge one spot to me.[5]

Three years after the ceremonial unveiling, Prince Albert died and the following year, 1862, Jenner disappeared from Trafalgar Square and reappeared in Kensington Gardens, where he remains today.

Jenner might have remained a relatively obscure figure in medical history if it had not been for the French chemist Louis Pasteur. In 1881, not long after Jenner's effigy was burned in the anti-vaccination campaign in Banbury, Oxfordshire, Pasteur was in London to attend the International

Medical Congress, where he would give an account of his exciting discovery that he could inoculate poultry to protect against a devastating disease known as 'chicken cholera'. He was examining the virus in his laboratory when he accidentally left some open to the air for a while. By chance, this attenuated the virus, so that when he injected it into chickens it protected them against a natural attack of the disease. It was a form of inoculation. Pasteur knew of Jenner's vaccine and decided to call his weakened strain of chicken cholera a vaccine, though it had no connection at all with cows or cowpox. And he went further than that. He concluded his address to the Medical Congress with a flourish:

> I cannot conclude, gentlemen, without expressing the great pleasure I feel at the thought that it is as a member of an International Medical Congress assembled in England that I make known the most recent results of vaccination upon a disease more terrible, perhaps, for domestic animals than small-pox is for man. I have given to vaccination an extension which science, I hope, will accept as homage paid to the merit, and to the immense services, rendered by one of the greatest men of England, Jenner. What a pleasure for me to do honour to this immortal name in this noble and hospitable city of London![6]

18

The Mystery of Immunity

Today, Jenner is often referred to as the 'father of immunology' because he inspired Pasteur. But really, Jenner had no more claim to that title than Lady Mary Wortley Montagu, or the Greek women inoculating in Constantinople, or Daniel Sutton. None of them knew anything of the micro-organisms that Pasteur and his contemporaries called 'germs'. As Sutton had written in *The Inoculator*:

> With respect to the peculiar miasma, or contagious essence, whatever it may be, should such a thing specifically and abstractedly exist (which as yet appears rather questionable) it is certainly of a nature too subtle, minute, and volatile, to be ascertained by any analysis yet known, nor have its contents been hitherto discovered by the help of our most perfect and compound microscopes.[1]

It took well over a century after the deaths of Sutton and Jenner for an accumulation of scientific investigation to gain some understanding of what had been going on medically when the inoculators and vaccinators sought to bring smallpox under control. While inoculation and vaccination appeared to be simple enough, the success they had was derived entirely from close observation of their effects on large numbers of patients. There was no science as such, as none of the pioneers knew anything about micro-organisms that caused diseases such as smallpox. And it was long time after the identification of 'germs', and the detective work that isolated the elements in them that caused specific infections, that it was understood that inoculation and vaccination worked because they triggered an immune response in the patient.

Anyone who caught smallpox 'naturally' was likely to have their immune system overwhelmed by the virus, which rapidly invaded the cells in their bodies where it could 'breed'. Whereas bacteria could survive without an animal host, smallpox could not propagate itself without invading a human body. When cells in the body detected the invader they set about destroying it. The hideous eruptions on the smallpox victim's body were a result of this epic battle between the immune system and the virus. Though he knew nothing of this, Sutton's method was to select lymph from a new pustule and inject only a small amount into the arm of his patient. It is now thought that he was successful because his inoculation triggered the immune system, giving it a kind of advance warning so that the body's defences could combat the virus before it took hold. The reason that inoculation conferred lifetime protection was that the immune system has a 'memory'. Another attack of the virus would alert killer cells which would rapidly root it out and destroy it.

Jenner's cowpox vaccine worked in the same way. It is an orthopox virus, one of a number which have an affinity with smallpox. The immune system would have detected certain proteins in the cowpox infection that were similar enough to trigger an immune response to smallpox. Successful vaccines were also derived from horse pox. It was because vaccine derived from cowpox was not an exact fit with smallpox virus that it did not last, and before long re-vaccination was needed to ensure life-long protection.

There was no way of analysing and comparing pox viruses in Jenner's day nor for a long time afterwards. But the new science of genetics made a remarkable discovery: the vaccines used around the world in a final push to eradicate smallpox were quite distinct from cowpox. They were closest to camel pox, but they had somehow evolved into quite a distinct virus that did not occur naturally.

An electron microscope powerful enough to detect smallpox virus was not available until the 1930s, by which time the disease was on the retreat in much of the industrialised world. A key to the success of the eradication programme launched in 1967 by the World Health Organization was the development of cleaner, more stable vaccines, though these were still mostly propagated through the injection of *vaccinia* into the scarified hides of calves. Modified vaccines had to be developed to survive in the hottest climates. As the areas where smallpox was endemic were identified, intensive propaganda campaigns were used to persuade anxious parents that their children's lives could be saved with a single injection. When outbreaks of 'wild' smallpox became rarer, villages were quickly quarantined to prevent the virus spreading.

What had begun with Lady Mary Wortley's discovery of a widely-practised folk medicine while living in Istanbul in the early eighteenth century had culminated more than 250 years later in the announcement by the World Health Organization that a once devastating epidemic illness was destroyed in the wild. Although Jenner is the one name associated worldwide with this unique medical achievement, every history of what we now call vaccination ought to have 1763 as a key date, the year Daniel Sutton as a young, unqualified country 'surgeon' began his practice in the Essex village of Ingatestone. The so-called Suttonian method of inoculation played a vital part in the acceptance of inoculation in sceptical populations the world over. Sutton also provided Jenner with a technique for introducing cowpox vaccination and a means of verifying whether or not it conferred immunity. There is no doubt that, without Sutton, vaccination would not have come about.

Sutton was undoubtedly a difficult, ungenerous character, intent on making a fortune from his skill rather than furthering the cause of medicine. He made no attempt to engage the medical authorities and frequently denigrated what he called the 'Faculty'. He was uneasy in 'polite society' and, as a *nouveau riche* he did not stay long in the elevated London world of Kensington Gore. Nothing characterised his sad desire for recognition better than his family coat of arms, which he bought for a few hundred pounds. Nevertheless, he *was* the Great Inoculator and deserves an honoured place in the history of the defeat of smallpox.

Postscript
Sutton's Family

We know something of Daniel Sutton's son, also Daniel, from a brief account of his rise and fall told in the little history of Ingatestone published in 1913. E.E. Wilde, the author of this document, assures the reader that much of his information came from one side of the family which kept its ties with Ingatestone. A reference is made to a Mrs Alex Campbell of Holland Park and 'many members of Daniel Sutton's family who helped to compile the history'. There were, he says, portraits of the children 'all with the sharp-cut nose that is so marked a feature in the father and the son, and most of them very good looking'. Sadly these pictures have not been found by recent research.

Wilde wrote:

As Maisonette remained in the hands of his descendants until quite recent years we may be permitted to follow shortly the fortunes of the family. Brought up to see the guineas flowing in with so little apparent effort, it is not surprising that young Daniel Sutton could never properly appreciate the value of money, and always made it go faster than it came. Put into law by his father, he started practice [*sic*] as a solicitor in Colchester; his heart, however, was not in his work, but, like the hearts of so many Essex men, away on the waters of our estuaries.[1]

In March 1790, Daniel married a Miss Anne Richardson and took a house at Wivenhoe on the River Colne, spending more time yachting than at his office in Colchester. Wilde wrote: 'He spent his money freely on boats and yachting and built a quay at Wivenhoe to which he gave his name. In one of his fast boats he is said to have brought to Wivenhoe, some say to London, the first news of victory at Waterloo.'[2] Daniel was made bankrupt on at least one occasion and yet was appointed Colchester Town Clerk. Though in a position in which he was expected to uphold the law, he became involved in smuggling, a popular line of business in Wivenhoe in the early nineteenth century.

Daniel's sister Frances married, in 1796, a Charles Campbell, who appears to have been financially sound. They had a large family, four daughters and two sons. It was the Campbell side of the family which inherited the portrait painted of her father when he was at the height of his fame. At one time they had some of Sutton's equipment, including his lancets, but attempts to trace them have failed. According to Wilde: 'As the years went by, children came to Daniel junior, but no wisdom: twice his brother-in-law Mr Charles Campbell, came to his rescue, but the third time the only offer of help was that of a passage to Tasmania for himself and his family, and this Sutton was compelled to accept.'[3]

Daniel's wife died before the exile to what was then known as Van Diemen's Land, leaving him with two daughters and a son. The older daughter, Eliza, took a post in Sydney, Australia, as a governess; there she married a Scotsman, Charles Cowper. They built a house they called Wivenhoe, had a large family and planted one of the earliest vineyards in New South Wales. When Charles was made governor of the state he was knighted and Eliza became Lady Cowper.

In 1832, when Daniel was 62 years old, he boarded the cargo ship the *Persian* with his younger daughter Charlotte and son Robert among the few passengers bound for Hobart, the main town on Van Diemen's Land.

It was a destination for convicted criminals sentenced to deportation. On the *Persian*, which was months at sea, Charlotte attracted the attention of the captain, Charles Friend. Not long after the ship docked in Hobart Town they were married. There is a census record of Daniel and his son Robert living in a house built of wood.

While his sister Eliza prospered in New South Wales, Robert came to an unfortunate end. Not much is known about his activities in Australia, but it seems likely that he got involved in the exploitation of the islands known as New Caledonia, to the east of Sydney, for sandalwood. English traders shipped it to China, where it was valued for its scent, and brought tea back to Australia. It was a risky enterprise for cannibalism was still widely practised. Catholic missionaries sent back reports of the crews of ships wrecked off the coast being killed and eaten. In a letter dated 'Sydney 1847', Father Jérôme Grange described his experiences for his friends who were parish priests in France. 'Of the Europeans who have flocked to this island are the English, who have come from Sydney seeking sandalwood. The natives have killed some of them and they are, they say, easier to kill than the New Caledonians. Besides they killed a man called Sutton whom they claimed was very good to eat.' There is no record of when Robert died. His father Daniel lived until the age of eighty-nine and was buried in Hobart in 1859.[4]

Notes

ACKNOWLEDGEMENTS

1. Essex Record Office, 1987.
2. Lord Rayleigh's Archives: letters in 1766, 8, 11, 22 April; 20, 26, 29 May; 6 June, Bamber Gascoyne to John Strutt.

PREFACE

1. Houlton, Robert, *Indisputable facts relative to the Suttonian art of inoculation. With observations on its discovery, progress, encouragement, opposition, etc.*, W. G. Jones, Dublin, 1768.

1 LADY MARY'S REVELATION

1. James Wharncliffe, ed., *The Letters of Lady Mary Wortley Montagu*, vol. 1, Henry G. Bohn, London, 1861, p. 308.
2. Wharncliffe, ed., *Letters of Lady Mary Wortley Montagu*, p. 328.
3. Maitland, Charles, *Mr Maitland's Account of Inoculating the Smallpox*, J. Downing, London 1722.
4. Ibid.
5. Ibid.
6. Ibid.
7. Ibid.
8. Ibid.
9. Genevieve Miller, 'Putting Lady Mary in her place: A discussion of historical causation', *Bulletin of the History of Medicine*, vol. 55, no.1, spring 1981, pp. 2–16.

2 SAVING THE QUALITY

1. *Daily Journal*, 17 June 1721.
2. Maitland, *Account of Inoculating the Smallpox*, 1722.
3. Ibid.
4. Wagstaffe, William, 'A letter to a friend showing the danger and uncertainty of inoculating the smallpox', Samuel Butler, London, 1722.

5. A Turky-Merchant, 'A Plain Account of the Inoculating of the Small Pox at Constantinople', *Flying Post*, September 1722.
6. Maitland, *Account of Inoculating the Smallpox*.

3 IS IT WORTH THE RISK?

1. *London Gazette*, 6–10 March 1722.
2. Sloane, Sir Hans and Birch, Thomas, 'An account of inoculation by Sir Hans Sloane, Bart. Given to Mr Ranby to be published, Annon 1736. Communicated by Thomas Birch, D.D. Secret R.S.', read 19 February 1756, *Philosophical Transactions*, vol. 49, 1755–6, pp. 516–20.
3. *Weekly Journal and British Gazetteer*, 30 November 1723.
4. A Turky-Merchant, 'A Plain Account of the Inoculating of the Small Pox at Constantinople', *Flying Post*, September 1722.
5. Thomas Nettleton, 'A letter from Dr Nettleton, Physician at Halifax in Yorkshire, to Dr Whitaker concerning the inoculation of the smallpox', *Philosophical Transactions of the Royal Society of London*, vol. 32, issue 370, 1 January 1723, pp. 35–48.
6. Nettleton, 'A letter from Dr Nettleton'.
7. James Jurin, 'A Letter to the Learned Caleb Cotesworth M.D., Fellow of the Royal Society of the College of Physicians and Physician to St Thomas's Hospital containing Comparison Between the Mortality of the Natural Small Pox and that Given INOCULATION by James Jurin', *Philosophical Transactions*, vol. 32, issue 374, 31 December 1723, https://doi.org/10.1098/rstl.1722.0038.
8. Nettleton, 'A letter from Dr Nettleton'.

4 A RURAL REVOLUTION

1. Nettleton, 'A letter from Dr Nettleton'.
2. James Carrick Moore, *The History of Smallpox*, Longman Hurst, London, 1815.
3. Thomas Dudley Fosbroke, *Biographical Anecdotes of Dr Jenner*, Berkely mss, Royal Collections Trust, 1821.
4. *Ipswich Journal*, 7 March 1767.
5. Houlton, *Indisputable facts*.
6. *Ispswich Journal*, 1757.
7. *Ipswich Journal*, 13 May 1766
8. William Woodville, *A History of the Inoculation of Smallpox in Great Britain*, vol.1, James Philips, 1796.
9. Lord Rayleigh's Archives: letter, 29 May 1766, Bamber Gascoyne to John Strutt.

5 A MOST SURPRISING FELLOW

1. Moore, *History of Smallpox*.
2. *Chelmsford Chronicle*, October 1764.
3. E.E. Wilde, *Ingatestone and the Essex Great Road with Fryerning*, Oxford University Press, London, 1913.
4. *Ipswich Journal*, November 1763.
5. *Chelmsford Chronicle*, May 1765.
6. *Ipswich Journal*, 6 July 1765.
7. Lord Rayleigh's Archives: letter, 29 May 1766, Bamber Gascoyne to John Strutt.

8. *Oxford Journal*, January 1766.
9. Moore, *History of Smallpox*.

6 SUTTON THE PARVENU

1. *Oxford Journal*, 7 June 1766.
2. Robert Houlton, *The practice of inoculation justified, a sermon preached at Ingatestone, Essex, 12 October 1766, in defence of inoculation.*
3. Butcher, Antony, 'Before Gore House', *Kensington Society Annual Report*, 2002, www.kensingtonsociety.org/wp-content/uploads/Annual-Report-2002.pdf
4. Daniel Sutton, *The Inoculator; or, Suttonian System of Inoculation Fully Set Forth in a Plain and Familiar Manner*, T. Gillett, London, 1796.
5. Wilde, *Ingatestone*.
6. *Ipswich Journal*, August 1767.
7. *Bath Chronicle and Weekly Gazette*, 19 January 1764.
8. Houlton, *The practice of inoculation justified*.
9. *Monthly Review*, vol. 36, 1767.
10. Houlton, *Indisputable facts*.
11. *Salisbury and Winchester Journal*, July 1767.
12. *Salisbury and Winchester Journal*, 13 July 1767.
13. *Oxford Journal*, 28 November 1767

7 SUTTON'S THUNDER STOLEN

1. George Baker (Physician to Her Majesty's Household), 'An inquiry into the merits of a method of inoculating which is now practiced in several Counties of England', *Monthly Review or Literary Journal*, vol. 35, 1766.
2. Thomas Ruston, *An Essay on Inoculation for the Small Pox Containing a Chymical Examination of Mr Sutton's Medicines*, London, 1768.
3. William Watson, *An Account of a Series of Experiments Instituted with a View of Ascertaining the Most Successful Method of Inoculating the Small-pox*, E. and C. Dilly, London, 1768.
4. Ibid.
5. Ibid.
6. Houlton, *Indisputable facts*.
7. Watson, *Account of a Series of Experiments*.
8. Richard Radcliffe and John James, *Letters of Richard Radcliffe and John James of Queens College Oxford 1755–1783*, edited by Margaret Evans, printed for the Oxford Historical Society by Clarendon Press, 1888.
9. Thomas Dimsdale, *The Present Method of Inoculating for the Small-pox*, Hertford, 1767.
10. Houlton, *Indisputable facts*.
11. Dimsdale, *The Present Method of Inoculating for the Small-pox*.

8 SUTTON MISSES THE BOAT

1. William Duncan et al., 'The Opinion of His Majesty's Physicians and Surgeons given Jan. 23, 1768, in regard to Messrs Sutton's practice in inoculation in consequence of a letter from Sir John Pringle, dated London, May 6, 1767, to Mr Brady at Brussels; and another from Count Kaunitz Rittburg, dated Vienna,

December 17, 1767 to Count Seilern, ambassador from the Empress Queen to the King of Great Britain', Signed Wm Duncan, Cl. Wintringham, R. Warren (Physicians to the king), J. Ranby, C. Hawkins, D. Middleton (Surgeons to the king), *Gentleman's Magazine*, vol. 38, February 1768, p. 75.

2. James Johnston Abraham, *Lettsom: His Life, Times, Friends and Descendants*, London, William Heinemann Medical Books, 1933.

3. Hester Thrale, *Thraliana: The Diary of Mrs Hester Lynch Thrale (Later Mrs Piozzi) 1776–1809*, edited by Katherine C. Balderston, vol. 1, *1776–1784*, 2nd edn, Oxford University Press, Oxford, 1951.

4. 'Anecdotes of Dr Dimsdale's inoculating the Czarina', *Town and Country Magazine* or *Universal Depository*, vol. 1, 1769, p. 309.

5. Thomas Dimsdale, *Tracts on Inoculation written and published at St Petersburg in the year 1768 by command of her Imperial Majesty the Empress of all the Russias with Additional Observations by Hon. Baron T. Dimsdale*, London, 1781.

6. Anthony Cross, *By the Banks of the Neva: Chapters from the Lives and Careers of the British in Eighteenth-century Russia*, Cambridge University Press, Cambridge, 1997.

7. Dimsdale *Tracts on Inoculation*.

8. J.S. Jenkins, 'The English inoculator, Jan Ingen-Housz', *Journal of the Royal Society of Medicine*, vol. 92, October 1999, pp. 534–7.

9 A SUTTONIAN IN AMERICA

1. J.L. Bell, 'Dr James Latham's inoculation franchise', Boston 1775 blog, October 2009, http://boston1775.blogspot.com/2009/10/dr-james-lathams-inoculation-franchise.html

2. William Lincoln, Section on James Latham in *History of Worcester, Massachusetts: From Its Earliest Settlement to 1836*, Moses D. Phillips and Co., Worcester, MA, 1837, p. 257.

3. *New York Gazette and Weekly Advertiser*, 13 August 1770.

4. Carl Bridenbaugh, *Cities in Revolt*, Alfred A. Knopf, New York, 1955.

5. Jeffrey Michael Weir, 'Account of James Latham' in *A Challenge to the Cause: Smallpox Inoculation in the Era of American Independence 1764 to 1781*, PhD dissertation, George Mason University, 2012.

6. *Essex Gazette*, 2 and 9 November 1773.

7. *Essex Gazette*, 8–15 March 1774.

8. *Connecticut Courant*, 30 August 1776.

10 AN IMPOSTER IN THE FAMILY

1. *London Evening Post*, 9 May 1771.

2. Michael Bennett, 'Curing and inoculating smallpox: The career of Simeon Worlock in Paris, Brittany and Saint-Domingue in the 1770s', *French History and Civilisation*, vol. 7, 2017, pp. 27–38.

3. Ibid.

4. https://www.findagrave.com/memorial/50067439/simeon-worlock

11 INOCULATION FOR THE INDUSTRIOUS POOR

1. Diana Crook, *Defying the Demon: Smallpox in Sussex*, Dale House Press, 2006.

2. *Gentleman's Magazine*, vol. LVIII, April 1788.

3. *Hampshire Chronicle*, 27 December 1773.
4. Ibid.
5. *Public Advertiser*, 9 February 1770.
6. *Newcastle Chronicle*, 20 October 1770.
7. Ibid.
8. *Public Advertiser*, 21 October 1772.
9. Ibid.
10. *Gazetteer and New Daily Advertiser*, 4 March 1772.
11. *Public Advertiser*, 27 October 1774.
12. *Gazetteer and New Daily Advertiser*, 20 September 1776.
13. *Hampshire Chronicle*, 24 January 1774.

12 SAVING THE NATION

1. John Haygarth, *An Inquiry How to Prevent the Small-pox: And Proceedings of a Society for Promoting General Inoculation at stated periods and preventing the natural small-pox, in Chester*, J. Monk, Chester, 1784.
2. John Haygarth, *A Sketch of a Plan to Exterminate the Casual Small-Pox from Great Britain*, J. Johnson, London, 1793.

13 SUTTON'S SWAN SONG

1. *Gazetteer and New Daily Advertiser*, 12 November 1776.
2. *Morning Post and Daily Advertiser*, Saturday 20 March 1784.
3. *Norfolk Chronicle*, 19 April 1788.
4. *Oxford Journal*, 12 April 1788.
5. Sutton, *The Inoculator*.
6. Ibid.
7. Ibid.
8. https://www.theguardian.com/science/2016/apr/26/morning-flu-jabs-could-save-thousands-of-lives-study-suggests
9. Sutton, *The Inoculator*.
10. Ibid.
11. Ibid.
12. Review of Sutton's book, *Critical Review or Annals of Literature*, vol. 21, 1797.

14 COWMANIA!

1. George Pearson, *An Inquiry Concerning the History of the Cow Pox*, J. Johnson, London, 1798.
2. John Baron, *The Life of Edward Jenner*, vol. 2, Henry Colburn, London, 1838.
3. Ibid.
4. *British Medical Journal*, 23 May 1896.
5. *Monthly Review*, 1 May 1804, p. 381.
6. Baron, *Life of Edward Jenner*.
7. Private communication from Professor Michael Bennett, 2019.
8. See John Z. Bowers, 'The Odyssey of Smallpox Vaccination', *Bulletin of the History of Medicine*, Vol. 55, No. 1 (Spring 1981), pp. 17–33.
9. *Bath Chronicle and Weekly Gazette*, 17 October 1799.
10. *Morning Advertiser*, 10 February 1807.

11. Arthur M. Silverstein, *A History of Immunology*, Academic Press, Boston and London, 1989.

15 JENNER'S DEBT TO SUTTON

1. *Derby Mercury*, 15 November 1798.
2. Silverstein, *A History of Immunology*.
3. Edward Jenner, *The Origin of the Vaccine Inoculation*, 1801.
4. Sutton, *The Inoculator*.
5. Ibid.
6. Edward Jenner, *An inquiry into the causes and effects of the Variolae Vaccinae, a disease discovered in some of the western counties of England, particularly Gloucestershire, and known by the name of the cow pox*, Sampson Low, London, 1798.
7. Ibid.
8. Ibid.
9. Baron, *Life of Edward Jenner*.
10. Ibid.
11. Rev. Edwin Sidney, *The Life of the Rev. Rowland Hill*, Seeley, Burnside and Seeley, London, 1834.
12. Letter to Dr Thomas Charles Morgan, 1 March 1809, in Edward Jenner, *Letters of Edward Jenner and Other Documents Concerning the Early History of Vaccination*, edited by Genevieve Miller, Johns Hopkins University Press, Baltimore, MD, 1983, p. 51.
13. Hansard, *House of Commons Debates 29 July 1807*, vol. 9, cc1007–15.

16 THE BATTLE FOR VACCINATION

1. *North Devon Journal*, 8 May 1828.
2. *Statesman*, 18 May 1821.
3. Ibid.
4. *Quarterly Review*, vol. 33, December 1825–March 1826.
5. Ibid.
6. John Cross, *A History of the Variolous Epidemic which occurred in Norwich in the year 1819 and destroyed 530 individuals with an estimate of the protection afforded by vaccination*, Burgess and Hill, London, 1820.
7. *Banbury Guardian*, 29 March 1877, p. 3.
8. *Aberdeen Press and Journal*, 28 March 1885.
9. *The Graphic*, 28 March 1885.
10. *A Report on Vaccination and its results based on evidence taken by The Royal Commission between 1880–1897*, New Sydenham Society, London, 1898.

17 SUTTON AND JENNER

1. *Gentleman's Magazine*, vol. 125, January–June 1819, p. 281.
2. *Gentleman's Magazine*, vol. 66, part 1, 1796.
3. See R.J. Davenport, J.P. Boulton, L. Schwarz, 'Urban inoculation and the decline of smallpox in eighteenth-century London', *The Economic History Review*, vol. 64, issue 4, 2011, pp. 1289–1314; P.E. Razzell, 'The decline of adult smallpox

mortality in eighteenth-century London: A commentary', *The Economic History Review*, vol. 64, issue 4, pp. 1315–35.
4. *Gentleman's Magazine*, vol 133, January–June 1823.
5. *Punch*, 22 May 1858.
6. Louis Pasteur, 'An address on vaccination in relation to chicken cholera and splenic fever', paper delivered at an International Medical Congress, *British Medical Journal*, 20 August 1881, pp. 283–4.

18 THE MYSTERY OF IMMUNITY

1. Sutton, *The Inoculator*.

POSTSCRIPT

1. Wilde, *Ingatestone*.
2. This turns out to be a family myth, see Brian Cathcart, *The News from Waterloo*, Faber & Faber, London, 2015.
3. Wilde, *Ingatestone*.
4. Fr Jérôme Grange to Fr Villerd, parish priest at Saint Jodard near Roanne and to Fr Nicoud, parish priest at Saint Clair near Condrieux, 18 September 1847, https://mariststudies.org/docs/Girard0661.

Bibliography

ARCHIVES

Lord Rayleigh's Archives
Oxford Brookes University Research Archive
Royal Collections Trust

NEWSPAPERS

Aberdeen Press and Journal
Banbury Guardian
Bath Chronicle and Weekly Gazette
British Medical Journal
Chelmsford Chronicle
Connecticut Courant
Critical Review of Annals of Literature
Daily Journal
Derby Mercury
Essex Gazette
Gazetteer and New Daily Advertiser
Gentleman's Magazine
Graphic
Guardian
Hampshire Chronicle
Ipswich Journal
London Evening Post
London Gazette
Monthly Review
Morning Advertiser
Morning Post and Daily Advertiser
New York Gazette and Weekly Advertiser
Newcastle Chronicle
Norfolk Chronicle

North Devon Journal
Oxford Journal
Public Advertiser
Punch
Quarterly Review
Salisbury and Winchester Journal
Statesman
Weekly Journal and British Gazetteer

'A letter from the same learned and ingenious gentleman concerning his farther progress in inoculating the Smallpox to Dr Jurin', *Philosophical Transactions*, vol. 32, issue 370, 1 January 1723.

A Report on Vaccination and its results based on evidence taken by The Royal Commission between 1880–1897, New Sydenham Society, London, 1898.

A Turky-Merchant, 'A Plain Account of the Inoculating of the Small Pox at Constantinople', *Flying Post*, September 1722.

Abraham, James Johnston, *Lettsom: His Life, Times, Friends and Descendants*, William Heinemann Medical Books, London, 1933.

'An authentic account of the state of inoculation at Ewell in Surrey', *Gentleman's Magazine*, vol. 36, 1766, pp. 413–14.

'Anecdotes of Dr Dimsdale's inoculating the Czarina', *Town and Country Magazine or Universal Depository*, vol. 1, 1769, p. 309.

Baker, George (Physician to Her Majesty's Household), 'An inquiry into the merits of a method of inoculating which is now practiced in several Counties of England', *Monthly Review or Literary Journal*, vol. 35, 1766.

Barnes, Diana, 'The public life of a woman of wit and quality: Lady Mary Wortley Montagu and the vogue for smallpox inoculation', *Feminist Studies*, vol. 38, no. 2, summer 2012, pp. 330–62.

Baron, John, *The Life of Edward Jenner*, 2 vols, Henry Colburn, London, 1838.

Bazin, Hervé, *Vaccination: A History from Lady Montagu to Jenner and Genetic Engineering*, John Libbey Eurotext Ltd, Esher, 2011.

Bell, J.L. 'Dr James Latham's inoculation franchise', Boston 1775 blog, October 2009, http://boston1775.blogspot.com/2009/10/dr-james-lathams-inoculation-franchise.

Bell, J.L., 'The "Suttonian Method" of fighting the Smallpox', Boston 1775 blog, October 2009, http://boston1775.blogspot.com/2009/10/suttonian-method-of-fighting-smallpox.html

Bennett, Michael, 'Jenner's ladies: Women and vaccination against smallpox in early nineteenth-century Britain', *History*, vol. 93, no. 4, October 2008, pp. 497–513.

Bennett, Michael, 'Inoculation of the poor against smallpox in eighteenth-century England', in *Experiences of Poverty in Late Medieval and Early Modern England and France*, ed. Anne M. Scott, Ashgate, Farnham, 2012.

Bennett, Michael, 'Curing and inoculating smallpox: The career of Simeon Worlock in Paris, Brittany and Saint-Domingue in the 1770s', *French History and Civilisation*, vol. 7, 2017, pp. 27–38.

Bennett, Michael, 'Vaccine's conquest of Napoleonic Europe', private communication, February 2019.

Booth, Christopher, 'John Haygarth (1740–1827)', *Journal of the Royal Society of Medicine*, vol. 107, no. 12, Dec. 2014, pp. 490–3.

Bowers, John Z., 'The Odyssey of Smallpox Vaccination', *Bulletin of the History of Medicine*, Vol. 55, No. 1 (Spring 1981), pp. 17–33.

Boylston, Arthur, 'William Watson's use of controlled clinical experiments in 1768', *Journal of the Royal Society of Medicine*, vol. 107, no. 6, 2014, pp. 246–8.

Boylston, Arthur, 'Smallpox inoculation: prelude to vaccination', *Hektoen International: A Journal of Medical Humanities*, vol. 11, no. 1, winter 2019.

Bridenbaugh, Carl, *Cities in Revolt*, Alfred A. Knopf, New York, 1955.

British History Online, 'Smallpox', in *A History of the County of Wiltshire*, vol. 5, London, Victoria County History, 1957, https://www.british-history.ac.uk/vch/wilts/vol5/pp318-347#h2-0004

Butcher, Antony, 'Before Gore House' (a history of Sutton House in Knightsbridge), *Kensington Society Annual Report*, 2002, www.kensingtonsociety.org/wp-content/uploads/Annual-Report-2002.pdf

Cathcart, Brian, *The News from Waterloo*, Faber and Faber, London, 2015.

Clendenning, Philip H., 'Dr Thomas Dimsdale and smallpox inoculation in Russia', *Journal of the History of Medicine and Sciences*, vol. 28, no. 2, April 1973, pp. 109–25.

Creighton, Charles, *Jenner and Vaccination: A Strange Chapter of Medical History*, Swan Sonnenschein & Co., London, 1889.

Creighton, Charles, *A History of Epidemics in Britain*, Cambridge University Press, Cambridge, 1891–1894 .

Crook, Diana, *Defying the Demon: Smallpox in Sussex*, Dale House Press, 2006.

Cross, Anthony, *By the Banks of the Neva: Chapters from the Lives and Careers of the British in Eighteenth-century Russia*, Cambridge University Press, Cambridge, 1997.

Cross, John, *A History of the Variolous Epidemic which occurred in Norwich in the year 1819 and destroyed 530 individuals with an estimate of the protection afforded by vaccination.* Burgess and Hill, London, 1820.

Dimsdale, Thomas, 'Memoirs of the Hon. Baron Dimsdale', *The European Magazine and London Review*, August 1802.

—— *The Present Method of Inoculating for the Small-pox*, Hertford, 1767.

—— *Thoughts on General and Partial Inoculations*, W. Owen, London, 1776.

—— *Tracts on Inoculation written and published at St Petersburg in the year 1768 by command of her Imperial Majesty the Empress of all the Russias with Additional Observations by Hon. Baron T. Dimsdale*, London, 1781.

Drew, Henry A., *Henry Knox and the Revolutionary War Trail in Western Massachusetts*, McFarland and Co., Jefferson, NC, 2012.

Duncan, William et al., 'The Opinion of His Majesty's Physicians and Surgeons given Jan. 23, 1768, in regard to Messrs Sutton's practice in inoculation in consequence of a letter from Sir John Pringle, dated London, May 6, 1767, to Mr Brady at Brussels; and another from Count Kaunitz Rittburg, dated Vienna, December 17, 1767 to Count Seilern, ambassador from the Empress Queen to the King of Great Britain', Signed Wm Duncan, Cl. Wintringham, R. Warren (Physicians to the king), J. Ranby, C. Hawkins, D. Middleton (Surgeons to the king). *Gentleman's Magazine*, vol. 38, February 1768.

Empson, John, 'Little honoured in his own country: statues in recognition of Edward Jenner', *Journal of the Royal Society of Medicine*, vol. 89, September 1996.

Fisher, Richard B., *Edward Jenner*, André Deutsch, London, 1991.

Fordyce, William, 'Account of general inoculation in Luton', letter in *Gentleman's Magazine*, April 1788, pp. 283–4.

Fosbroke, Thomas Dudley, *Biographical Anecdotes of Dr Jenner*, Berkely mss, Royal Collections Trust, 1821.

Frewen, Thomas, 'The practice and theory of Inoculation with an account of its success in a letter to a friend', London, 1749.

Gatrell, Vic, *The Hanging Tree: Execution and the English People*, Oxford University Press, Oxford, 1996.

Glynn, Ian and Glynn, Jennifer, *The Life and Death of Smallpox*, Profile Books, London, 2004.

Halsband, Robert, *The Life of Lady Mary Wortley Montagu*, Clarendon Press, Oxford, 1956.

——'New Light on Lady Mary Wortley Montagu's Contribution to Inoculation', *Journal of the History of Medicine and Allied Sciences*, Volume VIII, Issue October, October 1953, pp. 390–405.

Hansard, *House of Commons Debates 29 July 1807*, vol. 9, cc1007–15.

Haygarth, John, *An Inquiry How to Prevent the Small-pox: And Proceedings of a Society for Promoting General Inoculation at stated periods and preventing the natural small-pox, in Chester*, J. Monk, Chester, 1784.

Houlton, Robert, *The practice of inoculation justified, a sermon preached at Ingatestone, Essex, 12 October 1766, in defence of inoculation*.

Houlton, Robert, *Indisputable facts relative to the Suttonian art of inoculation. With observations on its discovery, progress, encouragement, opposition, etc.*, W. G. Jones, Dublin, 1768.

Huth, Edward, 'Quantitative evidence for judgments on the efficacy of inoculation for the prevention of smallpox: England and New England in the 1700s', *Journal of the Royal Society of Medicine*, vol. 99, issue 5, May 2006, 262–6.

Ipswich Journal, 'Dr Rodbard controversy with Daniel Sutton', *Ipswich Journal*, 14 February 1767, 28 February 1767.

Irvine, Sally, *Surgeons and Apothecaries in Suffolk: City Slickers and Country Bumpkins – Exploring Medical Myths*, PhD thesis, University of East Anglia, School of History, April 2011.

Jenkins, J.S., 'The English inoculator, Jan Ingen-Housz', *Journal of the Royal Society of Medicine*, vol. 92, October 1999, pp. 534–7.

Jenner, Edward, *A Continuation of Facts and Observations Relative to the Variolae Vaccinae or Cow Pox*, Sampson Low, London, 1800.

Jenner, Edward, *An inquiry into the causes and effects of the Variolae Vaccinae, a disease discovered in some of the western counties of England, particularly Gloucestershire, and known by the name of the cow pox*, Sampson Low, London, 1798, https://archive.org/details/b24759247/

Jenner, Edward, *Further Observations of the Variolae Vaccinae or Cow Pox*, Sampson Low, London, 1799.

Jenner, Edward, *Letters of Edward Jenner and Other Documents Concerning the Early History of Vaccination*, edited by Genevieve Miller, Johns Hopkins University Press, Baltimore, MD, 1983.

Jenner, Edward, *On the Origin of the Vaccine Inoculation*, N. Shury, London, 1801.

Jurin, James, 'A Letter to the learned Caleb Cotesworth M.D., Fellow of the Royal Society, of the College of Physicians and Physician to St Thomas's Hospital containing a comparison between the mortality of the Natural Small Pox and that given by INOCULATION by James Jurin', *Philosophical Transactions*, vol. 32, issue 374, 31 December 1723, https://doi.org/10.1098/rstl.1722.0038

Leadbeater, Rosemary A., 'Experiencing smallpox in eighteenth-century England', Oxford Brookes University Research Archive, 2015.

Lettsom, John Coakley, 'Memoirs of the Hon. Baron Dimsdale', *The European Magazine and London Review*, vol. 42, August 1802.

Lincoln, William, Section on James Latham in *History of Worcester, Massachusetts: From Its Earliest Settlement to 1836*, Moses D. Phillips and Co., Worcester, MA, 1837.

Macaulay, Thomas Babington, *The History of England from the Accession of James II*, vol. 4, Chapter Twenty, http://www.gutenberg.org/files/2613/2613-h/2613-h.htm

Maitland, Charles, *Mr Maitland's Account of Inoculating the Smallpox*, J. Downing, London, 1722.

May, Maisie, 'Inoculating the urban poor in the late eighteenth century', *British Journal for the History of Science*, vol. 30, no. 3, Student Papers, September 1997, pp. 291–305.

Mead, Richard, *A discourse on the Smallpox and Measles, by Richard Mead, Fellow of the Royal College of Physicians at London and Edinburgh and of the Royal Society and Physician to His Majesty*, John Brindley, London, 1748.

Miller, Genevieve, 'Smallpox inoculation in England and America: A reappraisal', *The William and Mary Quarterly*, vol. 13, no. 4, 1956, pp. 476–92.

Miller, Genevieve, *The Adoption of Inoculation for Smallpox in England and France*, University of Pennsylvania Press, Philadelphia, 1957.

Miller, Genevieve, 'Putting Lady Mary in her place: a discussion of historical causation', *Bulletin of the History of Medicine*, vol. 55, no. 1, spring 1981, pp. 2–16.

Monthly Review, The, vol. 36, 1767.

Moore, James Carrick, *The History of Smallpox*, Longman Hurst, London, 1815.

Nettleton, Thomas, 'A letter from Dr Nettleton, Physician at Halifax in Yorkshire, to Dr Whitaker concerning the inoculation of the smallpox', *Philosophical Transactions of the Royal Society of London*, vol. 32, issue 370, 1 January 1723, pp. 35–48.

Pasteur, Louis, 'An address on vaccination in relation to chicken cholera and splenic fever', paper delivered at an International Medical Congress, *British Medical Journal*, 20 August 1881.

Pearson, George, *An Inquiry concerning the history of the Cow Pox*, J. Johnson, London, 1798.

Power, Joseph, *Précis historique de la Nouvelle méthode d'inoculer La Petite Vérole; avec une Exposition abrégée de cette Méthode: Ouvrage Destiné à montrer comment elle s'est établie en Angleterre, les grands succès dont elle y a été suivie, & qu'elle est due incontestablement à M. Sutton*, Par M. Power Docteur en Médecine & instruit par L'Auteur même de sa Méthode, |A Amsterdam Et se trouve à Paris Chez Le Breton, premier Imprimeur ordinaire du Roi 1769.

Proceedings of the Old Bailey, London's Central Criminal Court, 1674 to 1913 https://www.oldbaileyonline.org/

Radcliffe, Richard and James, John, *Letters of Richard Radcliffe and John James of Queens College Oxford 1755–1783*, edited by Margaret Evans, printed for the Oxford Historical Society by Clarendon Press, 1888.

Razzell, Peter, *Edward Jenner's Cowpox Vaccine: The History of a Medical Myth*, 2nd edn, Caliban Books, Firle, 1980.

Razzell, Peter, *The Conquest of Smallpox: The Impact of Inoculation on Smallpox Mortality in Eighteenth-century Britain*, 2nd edn, Caliban Books, Firle, 2003.

Rees, Abraham (ed.) 'Inoculation', in *The Cyclopaedia or Universal Dictionary of Arts, Sciences and Literature*, 39 vols, vol. 19, Longman Hurst, London, 1819.

Review of Sutton's book, *Critical Review or Annals of Literature*, vol. 21, 1797.

Review of Sutton's book, *Analytical Review of History of Literature, Domestic and Foreign*, vol. 25, 1797.

Rusnock, Andrea, 'Historical context and the roots of Jenner's discovery', *Human Vaccines and Immunotherapies*, vol. 12, no. 8, 2016.

Ruston, Thomas, *An Essay on Inoculation for the Small Pox Containing a Chymical Examination of Mr Sutton's Medicines*, 3rd edn, E. and C. Dilly, London, 1768.

Sidney, Edwin, *The Life of the Rev. Rowland Hill*, Seeley, Burnside and Seeley, London, 1834.

Silverstein, Arthur M., *A History of Immunology*, Academic Press, Boston and London, 1989.

Sloane, Sir Hans and Birch, Thomas, 'An account of inoculation by Sir Hans Sloane, Bart. Given to Mr Ranby to be published, Annon 1736. Communicated by Thomas Birch, D.D. Secret R.S.', read 19 February 1756, *Philosophical Transactions*, vol. 49, 1755–6, pp. 516–20.

Smith, J.R., *The Speckled Monster, Smallpox in England 1670–1970 with Particular Reference to Essex*, Essex Record Office, Chelmsford, 1987.

Smith, Kendall A., 'Edward Jenner and the smallpox vaccine', *Frontiers in Immunology*, vol. 2, 14 June 2011.

South, Mary, *The Inoculation Book 1774–1783*, Southampton Records Series, vol. 47, University of Southampton, 2014.

Stearns, Raymond Phineas and Pasti Jr, George, 'Remarks upon the introduction of inoculation for smallpox in England', *Bulletin of the History of Medicine*, vol. 24, no. 2, March–April 1950, pp. 103–22.

Sutton, Daniel, *The Inoculator; or, Suttonian System of Inoculation Fully Set Forth in a Plain and Familiar Manner*, T. Gillett, London, 1796.

Thrale, Hester, *Thraliana: The Diary of Mrs Hester Lynch Thrale (Later Mrs Piozzi) 1776–1809*, edited by Katherine C. Balderston, vol. 1, *1776–1784*, 2nd edn, Oxford University Press, Oxford, 1951.

Thurston, L. and Williams, G., 'An examination of John Fewster's role in the discovery of smallpox vaccination', *Journal of the Royal College of Physicians*, vol. 45, 2015, pp. 173–9.

Tunis, Barbara, 'Dr James Latham (*c.* 1734–1799): pioneer inoculator in Canada', *Canadian Bulletin of Medical History*, vol. 1, no. 1, spring 1984, pp. 1–11 (published online 11 November 2016).

Turk, J.L. and Allen, Elizabeth, 'The influence of John Hunter's inoculation practice on Edward Jenner's discovery of vaccination against smallpox', *Journal of the Royal Society of Medicine*, vol. 83, April 1990.

Valentine, Sylvia, 'A forgotten Scottish hero?' (biography of Charles Maitland), *Kirk Notes*, April 2018, pp. 8–10, http://www.methlickparishchurch.co.uk/Notes.

Wagstaffe, William, 'A letter to a friend showing the danger and uncertainty of inoculating the smallpox', Samuel Butler, London, 1722.

Watson, William, *An Account of a Series of Experiments Instituted with a View of Ascertaining the Most Successful Method of Inoculating the Small-pox*, J. Nourse, London, 1768.

Weir, Jeffrey Michael, 'Account of James Latham' in *A Challenge to the Cause: Smallpox Inoculation in the Era of American Independence 1764 to 1781*, PhD dissertation, George Mason University, 2012.

Wharncliffe, James, ed., *The Letters and Works of Lady Mary Wortley Montagu*, vol. 1, Henry G. Bohn, London, 1861.

Wilde, E.E., *Ingatestone and the Essex Great Road with Fryerning*, Oxford University Press, London, 1913.

Williams, Gareth, *Angel of Death*, Palgrave Macmillan, Basingstoke, 2010.

Woodville, William, *A History of the Inoculation of Smallpox in Great Britain*, vol. 1, James Phillips, London, 1796.

Index

Relationships in parentheses are to Daniel Sutton. Unattributed headings and subheadings refer to Daniel Sutton.

'Lady Mary' in subheadings is Lady Mary Wortley Montagu.

Abraham, James Johnston 156
Acts of Parliament 152–3 see also
    Parliament
Adventure (ship) 127
Africa 27, 90
Albert, Prince 160
Alcock, John 11, 13–14, 19
Amelia, Princess 21
America 79–85, 128–9 see also United States
Amyand, Claudius 21, 27
Année Litteraire, l' 88
Antigua 54–5, 87, 92
Asclepiades 53
Aubert, Antoine 126–7
Austro-Hungarian Empire 125

Baker, Sir George 55, 59–60
Banbury 152, 160
Baron, John 127, 133–4, 140–1, 159
Barts (Hospital) 15
Bedford Street, Bloomsbury 142
Berkeley, Earl of 137
Berkeley, Gloucestershire 119, 136, 142,
    159
Berlin 68–9, 149
blood letting 5–6, 31–2, 117
Bloomsbury 112–13
Board of Guardians, Norwich 150
Boston (US) 27, 79
Boulogne 127
Boylston, Zabediel Dr 27
Breda, Netherlands 76

Broad Street, New York 81
Buhot, Inspector 88
Bury St Edmunds 36
Butcher, Anthony 52
Bute, John Stuart Earl of 95
Bute, Lady 7 see also Wortley Montagu,
    Mary (daughter)

Café Baptiste, Paris 88
calomel 60–1
camelpox 164
Campbell, Alex 166
Campbell, Charles 167
Canary Islands 128
Capell, Dr 33
capital punishment 10–11
Caribbean 86, 87, 89 see also Antigua;
    Jamaica; West Indies
Caroline, Princess 8, 9, 17, 19, 20–1
Carro, Jean de 124–6
Castle Auckland 93
'Castle Pox' 82
Catherine the Great 71–5, 77
cattle
    dairy cattle 119
    infecting with smallpox 129
    inoculation precedent and 133
    Jenner's breakthrough xiii
    Sacco in Lombardy 125
    Sutton unfamiliar with 136
    see also cowpox
Cauthrey, John 12, 13

Central Committee of Vaccination (France) 127
Central Criminal Court (Old Bailey) 10
Charlotte Street, London 113
Chatham, Earl of 52
Chelmsford 43, 55
Cheltenham 101, 159
Chertsey 54
Chester 106–11
Chichester 27, 28
chicken cholera 161
Child's Coffee House 15
Chippenham 22
Chiswell, Sarah 2
Christ's Hospital, London 13, 15
Christ's Hospital Buildings, Hertford 18
church, attitude of 95–6, 141
Cirencester 32
Clissold, Rev Dr 32
Coaster's Harbour (US) 105
coat of arms 53–5, 113, 114, 165
Coke, Lady Mary 52
Colchester 39, 166, 167
College of Heralds 53
Colne, River 167
Compulsory Vaccination Acts 153
confluent smallpox xiii *see also* smallpox
Constantinople (later Istanbul) 3, 5, 16–17, 162, 164
Continental Congress (US) 84
'cool treatment' 60, 67
Copenhagen 149
Council of the Five Nations (Indigenous Americans) 124
Cowper, Charles 167
cowpox
    description of 137
    Jenner on 121, 134
    Jenner's name for xiii
    London dairies 122–3
    smallpox and 119, 130, 137–8, 143, 163
Cremona 125
Cross, John 149–51
cuckoos 119, 140
Cumberland, Duke of 22, 72

dairies 122–3
dairy maids 133–5
Darnley, Lord 22
Davies, Revd Thomas 93–5
Dawson, John 111
Dimsdale, Nicholas 72, 75

Dimsdale, Dr Thomas 64–8, 73–8
    copies Sutton 79
    'Dimsdation' 84
    riches in Russia 87
    Sir John Pringle and Russia 72
    Society for the Inoculation of the Poor and 109
    and dispensaries for the poor 109
Dorchester, Evelyn Pierrepont, Marquess of 1
'Dr James's Powder' 47
Dublin 56
Duke, Mr 57
Duncombe, Thomas 160

East Sussex 94
Edinburgh 73, 77, 124
Elgin, Lady 125
Elgin, Lord 125
engrafting xiv, 2, 3–4, 12–13, 28 *see also* inoculation; smallpox
Evans, Richard 11, 13, 19
execution 10–11

Feodorovna, Empress Maria of Russia 126
Ferdinand IV (Naples and Sicily) 64
Ferguson, Dr 148
Final Report, 1896 Royal Commission report on vaccination 158
Florida 128
Fort George, Upper Canada 124
Fosbroke, Thomas Dudley 32, 33
Foundling Hospital, London 61–2, 76, 79, 94
Framlingham Hall 113
France 88–90, 126–8
Franklin, Benjamin 77
fresh air
    Daniel Sutton encourages 40, 48
    Dimsdale follows Sutton 75
    Dimsdale queries 65
    other doctors' methods 31
    Sir George Baker's puzzlement 60
    Worlock in Paris 89
Friend, Charles 168

gallows 10–11
Gascoyne, Bamber ix, 44–7, 59
genetics 163
Geneva, University of 126
George I, King 8, 9, 21, 52, 110
George II, King 12, 93
George III, King 110

Germany 125
'germs' xii, 116, 162
Gibraltar 126
Gloucester Cathedral 159
Gloucestershire 121, 123, 133, 138
Glynde, East Sussex 93–5
Golden Horn 2
Goodge Street, London 100, 101
Grange, Father Jérôme 168
Gray's Inn Road 122
Great Barrington, Massachusetts Bay 84
Great East Road 39, 69
Great Russell Street, Bloomsbury 142
Greek women inoculators 3, 33, 162
Grove House 52
Guildhall, Winchester 97
Guy's Hospital 124

Haiti 89
Halifax (Yorkshire) 24, 25, 28
Hapsburgs 69
Harrison, Elizabeth 10–11, 18–19
Hart Street (later Theobalds Road) 142, 156
Harwich 39
Haverford West 28
Haygarth, John
    Chester infirmary 106
    Chester Smallpox Society 107
    Chester's Rules of Prevention 109, 110
    on compulsory inoculation 111
    immunity from smallpox, views of 135
    inoculation of children 147
    research on transmission of smallpox
        116
Hertford 64–5, 78
Hill, Revd Rowland 141
Hobart, Tasmania 167–8
Hodgson, William 93–4
Holbrow, Mr 32
horsepox 163
Houlton, Revd Robert xv, 51–2, 54–6, 141
Houlton, Robert Jnr 35, 55, 56, 64, 67
humours, theory of 31
Hungary 125
Hunter, John 119

Ilchester, Earl of xv, 55, 56
Iles, Anne 78
immune system x, 115, 118, 163
immunisation 27
immunity 135–8, 163–4
    after smallpox 13, 17, 19, 32
    for life xiv, 146, 154
    Foundling Hospital staff 61

immunology xii, 131, 132, 162
Industrial Revolution 158
infectious diseases xii, xiii, 33
Ingatestone, Essex
    History of Ingatestone and the Great Essex
        Road 41, 53, 166
    Revd Houlton xv
    Sutton's home in 50
    Sutton's practice in ix, 39, 64
    warned against Sutton 42
Ingen-Housz, Jan 76–8, 79, 87
inoculation
    banned by Parliament 151
    becomes more acceptable 48
    'cool treatment' 60, 67
    early brutal methods 31–2
    fierce opposition to xiv–xv
    goes into decline 29
    meat-free diets 60, 62, 74
    mornings better than afternoons
        115–16
    public prefer over vaccination 145–6
    success rates 27–9
    vaccination seen as improvement on
        132–3, 140
International Medical Congress 160–1
Ipswich 158
Ipswich Arms and Chequers Inn 39
Ipswich hospital 157
Ireland 56
Isle of Wight 56
Istanbul see Constantinople

Jamaica 12, 56
Jefferson, Thomas 123
Jenner, Edward 121–30, 133–43
    background and character 119
    BMJ commemorative issue 123
    compulsory vaccination and its
        difficulties 111
    cowpox and smallpox 130, 134, 137–8
    dairy maids myth 133–5
    death 158–9
    effigies burned and hanged 152, 153,
        160
    faulty research 121
    inoculated as a boy 32–3, 65
    Pasteur tribute 161, 162
    Russian Empress thanks 126
    stipend from Parliament 142–4
    Sutton and 129, 136, 141–3, 156, 164
    worldwide fame xii, 145
Jenner, Henry 129, 139, 159
Jesty, Benjamin 143

Johnson, Dr Samuel 71
Jurin, Dr James 26–8

Keith, Dr 6
Kensington (Gore) 52
Kensington Gardens 160
Kensington Palace 52
Kenton, Suffolk 33, 40
Kingston upon Hall, Evelyn Pierrepont, Duke of 1

Latham, James 79–85
Latham family 85
Leeds 28
Leicester anti-vaccination protest153
Leicester Street, London 54, 101, 112
Leiden University 124
Lettsom, John Coakley 109
Lisle Street, London 112
Livingston Manor, New York 85
Lombardy 125
London Smallpox Hospital 127
Long Island 105
Lugano 124
Luton 95–6

Macaulay, T.B. xii
Macclesfield 28
Magdalen College, Oxford 56
Maisonette (house) 44, 50, 166
Maitland, Charles 2–6, 12–15, 18, 21, 26
Maldon, Essex 48–9
Malta 126
Marble Arch 10
Marblehead, Massachusetts 82
Marcet, Alexander 124
Maria Josepha (of Austria) 69
Maria Theresa, Empress (Austria) 69, 77
Marshall, William Calder 160
Massachusetts Bay 84
Massey, Isaac 15
Mather, Cotton 27–8
mercury 61, 83
Merret, Joseph 137
microscopes xii, 116, 164
Milan 125
Mohawk People 85, 124
Montagu, Lady Mary Wortley *see* Wortley Montagu, Lady Mary
Monticello 123
Montreal 80, 81
Moor (servant) 45–7
Moore, James Carrick 31, 40, 48
Morgan, Dr Thomas Charles 142

Moscow 126
Mozart, Leopold 69, 75–6
Mozart, Wolfgang Amadeus 69, 75–6
Mussin-Pushkin, Count 71

Napoleon Bonaparte 126, 127, 128
National Anti-compulsory Vaccination League 153, 154
National Health Service and vaccination 155
National Vaccine Establishment 147
Nelmes, Sarah 139
Nettleton, Thomas 24–31
Nevis (Caribbean) 12
New Caledonia 168
New Jersey 90
New York 81, 84, 85, 105
Newcastle upon Tyne 99, 100
Newgate Gaol 8–19, 26, 77, 79, 110
Newport, Rhode Island 104
North, Mary 12, 13
Norwich 149–150

Old Bailey 10, 12, 18
Ottomans 3, 125
Oxford Journal 47, 57, 113
Oxford Street 10

Paris 77, 86–90, 127, 129
Parliament xii, 142–3, 145, 151, 152–3
Pasteur, Louis 81, 162
Pearson, Doctor George 123, 143
Peel, Robert 159
Pera, Constantinople 2
Perceval, Spencer 143
Père Lachaise cemetery, Paris 88
Persian (ship) 167–8
Philadelphia 81, 84
Phipps, James (first vaccination 1796) 139, 142, 159
Pickering, Timothy 83
Pierrepont, Evelyn 1
Pitt, William 52
Poland 125
Poland Street, Soho 20
Poor Law Guardians 151
Pope, Alexander 1
population rise ix, 73
Power, Joseph 87
Priestley, Joseph 77
Pringle, Sir John 72, 76–8
Prussia 68–9, 126, 149
Puerto Rico 128
purging 5–6, 14, 22, 31–2, 61

quackery 47
Quakers 66, 109
quarantine 104, 107, 148, 164
Quebec 79–81, 85

Radcliffe, Revd Richard 65
Rathbone Place 101
Rayleigh, Lord ix
Razzell, Dr Peter ix, 157
Rhode Island 104–5
Richardson, Anne (daughter-in-law) 167
Rigby, Dr 150
Rodbard, John 33–5
Rolt, Edward 22
Rolt, Miss 22
Royal College of Physicians 110, 143, 148
Royal College of Surgeons 147
Royal Commission on Vaccination (1896)
    154, 158
Royal Society 26, 27, 77, 119
rue de la Comédie Française, Paris 88
Rules of Prevention (Chester Smallpox
    Society) 107–10
Russia 71–3
Ruston, Thomas 60–1
Ryegate (Reigate) 94

Sacco, Dr Luigi 125
Saint-Domingue 89–90, 92
Salem, Massachusetts 82–3
Salisbury 57
Salonika 125
sandalwood 168
Sartine, Antoine de 87–8, 89
Schönbrunn palace 76
Seilern, Count 69
Selectmen 82
Sheehy, Dr 88–9
Shepton Mallet 55
Shuttleworth, Dr (brother-in-law) 81
Sievier, William 159
Silverstein, Arthur 131, 132
slave, knowledge of inoculation 27
slave trade 89, 90, 92
Sloane, Sir Hans 9, 12, 18, 21
smallpox
    effects of xii–xiii
    eradication of, 155
    immune system and virus battle 163
Smallpox Hospital, St Pancras 122, 127,
    130
Smallpox Society, Chester 107–8, 111
Smith, John ix, 157
Smith, Mr Jnr 97–8

Society for the Inoculation of the Poor in
    their own Homes 109
Society of Medicine (Paris) 127
South America 128
Southampton 102
Southampton Street, Bloomsbury 113
Spain 126, 128
St Edmundbury 158
St George's Hospital, Hyde Park Corner 123
St Mary the Virgin, Berkeley 159
St Marylebone 123
St Petersburg 71–5, 126
Steigerthal, Dr 18
Strutt, John 44–5, 46, 47
Stuart, John Earl of Bute 95
Stuart, Hon. Revd William 95–7
Suffolk 36
Sutton, Charlotte (granddaughter) 167
Sutton, Daniel
    argument with father over methods 37–8
    birth of xiii
    brother Robert's inoculation 34–5
    builds chapel 50–1
    called 'illiterate and ignorant' 57
    coat of arms 53–4, 113, 114, 165
    combative nature 55, 56–8, 165
    death 156
    death of wife 92
    earnings 41, 44, 49
    experiments 116–18
    foreign interest in 68–72
    franchise system 44, 56–7
    growing latter-day interest in 157
    importance of fresh air 40, 48,
    Jenner and 129, 136, 141–3, 156, 164
    King's physicians on 70
    marriage 54
    rough and ready nature 70–1
    Royal Commission on Vaccination
        considers his work 154
Sutton, Daniel (son) 92, 166–8
Sutton, Eliza (granddaughter) 167, 168
Sutton, Frances Dominicittie (daughter)
    92, 167
Sutton, Rachel (wife) 54–5, 86, 92
Sutton Robert (brother) 34–7, 87
Sutton, Robert (father) 34–8
    death 113
    sole inventor claims 101
Sutton, Robert (grandson) 167, 168
Sutton, Sarah (mother) 113
Sutton, William (brother) 80–1, 100–1, 113
Sutton family 37, 44, 64, 113
Sutton House 52–4, 86, 99, 101, 112, 136

Suttonian inoculation
  Jenner's vaccination impossible without 138
  superseded by vaccination 129–30
  vaccinators paint grim picture of 151
Swan public house, Ingatestone 43–4
Sydenham, Dr Thomas 60, 67
Sydney (Australia) 167
Symons family 24

Tasmania 167
Temple Stairs, London 11
Tenerife 128
Thames, River 11
Thetford 113
Thorsby Hall 1
Thrale, Hester Lynch 71
Timoni, Dr Emanuel 3
Tompion, Ann 11, 13, 14
Tompion, Mr 11
Trafalgar Square 160
Trenton, New Jersey 91
Trevor, Rt Revd Richard 93–4, 95
Trinity College, Cambridge 26
Tunbridge Wells 94
Turkish inoculation 2–5, 125
  Cotton Mather learns about 27
  Lady Mary's newspaper article 16–17
  Sutton's approach and 33
Tyburn 10

United States 123–4, 160 see also America

vaccination 118–31
  advantages over inoculation 146–7
  discovery of 119–20
  English and European attitudes to, a comparison 148–9
  free national scheme 151
  an improvement on inoculation 132–3, 140
  international demand for 122–9
  Pasteur's use of the term vaccine 161
  protests and riots against 152–4, 160
  re-vaccination necessary 152, 163
Vaccination Acts 151–2
Vaccinoff 126
Van Zwanenberg, David 157
variolae vaccinae see cowpox
variolation xii

Vauxhall 54, 112
Vesey, Captain 127
Victoria, Queen 160
Vienna 69, 70, 71, 75–6, 77–8, 124
Virginia 56, 123
Voltaire 73

Wagstaffe, William 15–16, 17, 23
Wakley, Thomas 151
Wallis, Mrs 45–6
Wandsworth 54
War of Austrian Succession 76
Waterhouse, Dr Benjamin 104–5
Watkinson, John 109
Watson, William 61–4
West Indies 19, 50 see also Antigua; Caribbean; Jamaica
Westley, Rachel (née Worlock) 54–5 see also Sutton, Rachel
Westley, William 54–5
Wharncliffe, Lord 6–7
Whiting, Dr William 84
Wilde, E.E. 41, 53, 166, 167
William Augustus, Prince 21–2 see also Cumberland, Duke of
Winchester 97, 99
Wivenhoe, Essex 167
'Wivenhoe' (house) 167
Woodbridge, Suffolk 33
Woodville, William 37, 41, 122–3, 127
Worcester, Massachusetts 81
World Health Organisation (WHO) 164
Worlock, Rachel (later Rachel Westley; Rachel Sutton) 54–5
Worlock, Simeon Jnr 89, 90–1
Worlock, Simeon Snr (father-in-law) x, 54, 86–90
Wortley Montagu, Edward Jnr 1, 2, 3, 4
Wortley Montagu, Edward Snr 1, 2
Wortley Montagu, Lady Mary 1–8
  anonymous newspaper article 16–17, 22–3
  Greek ladies in Turkey 33
  Revd Houlton praises xv, 51–2
  on Turkish inoculation 30
Wortley Montagu, Mary (daughter, later Lady Bute) 3, 4–7

York 149
Yorkshire 27
Yucatan 128